DIAGNOSIS

DIAGNOSIS

A Guide for Medical Trainees

Ashley Graham Kennedy, PhD

OXFORD
UNIVERSITY PRESS

OXFORD
UNIVERSITY PRESS

Oxford University Press is a department of the University of Oxford. It furthers
the University's objective of excellence in research, scholarship, and education
by publishing worldwide. Oxford is a registered trade mark of Oxford University
Press in the UK and certain other countries.

Published in the United States of America by Oxford University Press
198 Madison Avenue, New York, NY 10016, United States of America.

Library of Congress Cataloging-in-Publication Data
Names: Kennedy, Ashley Graham, author.
Title: Diagnosis: a guide for medical trainees / Ashley Graham Kennedy.
Description: New York : Oxford University Press, [2021] |
Includes bibliographical references and index.
Identifiers: LCCN 2021008091 (print) | LCCN 2021008092 (ebook) |
ISBN 9780190060411 (paperback) | ISBN 9780190060435 (epub) |
ISBN 9780190060442 (online)
Subjects: MESH: Diagnosis | Diagnostic Techniques and Procedures |
Clinical Decision-Making | Physician-Patient Relations
Classification: LCC RT48 (print) | LCC RT48 (ebook) | NLM WB 141 |
DDC 616.07/5—dc23
LC record available at https://lccn.loc.gov/2021008091
LC ebook record available at https://lccn.loc.gov/2021008092

DOI: 10.1093/med/9780190060411.001.0001

This material is not intended to be, and should not be considered, a substitute for medical or other
professional advice. Treatment for the conditions described in this material is highly dependent
on the individual circumstances. And, while this material is designed to offer accurate information
with respect to the subject matter covered and to be current as of the time it was written, research
and knowledge about medical and health issues is constantly evolving and dose schedules for
medications are being revised continually, with new side effects recognized and accounted for
regularly. Readers must therefore always check the product information and clinical procedures with
the most up-to-date published product information and data sheets provided by the manufacturers
and the most recent codes of conduct and safety regulation. The publisher and the authors make no
representations or warranties to readers, express or implied, as to the accuracy or completeness of
this material. Without limiting the foregoing, the publisher and the authors make no representations
or warranties as to the accuracy or efficacy of the drug dosages mentioned in the material. The
authors and the publisher do not accept, and expressly disclaim, any responsibility for any liability,
loss, or risk that may be claimed or incurred as a consequence of the use and/or application of any of
the contents of this material.

1 3 5 7 9 8 6 4 2

Printed by Marquis, Canada

CONTENTS

PREFACE

In late June of 2018, Oxford University Press contacted me to ask if I would be interested in writing a book on medical uncertainty, a topic I had written several articles on previously. While honored by their request, I told them that I would rather write a book about the practice of medical *diagnosis*, which is a topic that I had been thinking and writing about for six years at that time. After finishing a dissertation on scientific models and representation at the University of Virginia in 2012, I had accepted a two-year postdoctoral position at the University of South Carolina in order to devote my time to a study of my newly found passion: the philosophy of medicine. On the first day of my post-doc, I had set myself to the task of mapping out a reading plan of all of the available philosophy of medicine literature on medical diagnosis. I figured that because diagnosis was the starting point of medicine, it should also be the starting point of my postdoctoral reading. *Five minutes later,* I realized that there was essentially no philosophical literature on diagnosis, and no systematic evaluation of the concepts involved in the process of diagnosing a patient. What a shock! Although there was plenty of interesting work going on in the philosophy of medicine, at the time it was al-most exclusively focused on the evaluation of medical treatments. Most of the medical literature, on the other hand, was devoted either to the specific question of how to evaluate medical diagnostics or to the issue of heuristics and bias in diagnostic practice. I could not find any work—either philosophical or medical—that examined the concepts involved in diagnostic practice as a whole. So I began to study, and to write on, these issues on my own, drawing on my scientific background and philosophical training as well as in-clinic observations at Columbia University Medical Center, while simul-taneously teaching these topics to premedical students, medical students, and medical residents at the University of South Carolina and Florida Atlantic University.

Now, nearly eight years later, this book is the result of that work. I do not pretend to have written a book that addresses all of the philosophical or conceptual issues inherent in the practice of clin-ical diagnosis: The reader will notice that there are many I have left untouched. However, the topics that I have chosen to address are all theoretically important ones that also have direct relevance to actual, everyday clinical practice. While I hope that what follows will be of interest to all medical practitioners, medical students, philosophers of medicine, and patient advocates, I have primarily written it with an audience of medical trainees—interns, residents, and fellows—in mind. As such, philosophers will notice that I do not always give a full defense of the philosophical arguments I pre-sent. Instead, I leave that to future work. I hope that in what follows, you will find a work worth reading.

Tequesta, Florida
December 2020

ACKNOWLEDGMENTS

I have many to thank for making the writing of this book possible. First, I thank Miriam Solomon, who years ago, after reading a draft of one of my first articles on diagnosis, remarked that, "It wasn't an article at all, but rather a book." I have reminded myself of these words on many occasions, and they have served as motivation to see this project through to completion. Thank you Miriam, for your encouragement and support. I am also grateful to Bryan Cwik, Dusty Hardman, Sarah Malanowski, Mark Tunick, and Donna Ray, who generously volunteered to read parts of or, in some cases, the entirety of the manuscript prepublication. Their comments have undoubtedly made the book better than it would have been otherwise.

Parts of three previously published articles and two book chapters appear in Chapters 2–5. Chapter 2 contains material from "Evaluating Diagnostic Tests," published in *Journal of Evaluation in Clinical Practice* in 2015. Chapter 3 expands upon material from a book chapter published in the 2016 *Routledge Companion to Philosophy of Medicine*, called "Medical Decision Making." Chapter 4 elaborates on material from "Managing Diagnostic Uncertainty," which was published in *Journal of Evaluation in Clinical Practice* in 2015, as well as material from "Differential Diagnosis and the Suspension of Judgment," which appeared in *Journal of Medicine and Philosophy* in 2013. Chapter 5 contains material from a forthcoming chapter, "Imaging, Representation and Diagnostic Uncertainty," in *Philosophy of Advanced Medical Imaging* (Springer, 2020). All of the other material in this book is new.

And finally, I am forever grateful for my family—my husband Bobby and my two sons, Micaiah and Kai—who never fail to support me in all of my endeavors—academic or otherwise. I love you.

Introduction

I.1. OVERVIEW

Philosophers have been writing about the practice of medicine for some time. In particular, in recent years, philosophers of medicine have been asking, and seeking to answer, questions concerning both the epistemology and the metaphysics of medical practice. Epistemology, generally speaking, is the philosophical study of the nature and extent of knowledge either globally or in a given domain, whereas metaphysics (although notoriously difficult to define) is generally understood to be the study of the fundamental nature of reality, or what it is that exists. These questions, as they pertain to medicine, are not only philosophically interesting but also practically relevant. Most of the recent epistemological work in philosophy of medicine has been concerned with medical treatments and interventions, specifically with questions about efficacy, evidence, and extrapolation regarding their evaluation. Recent metaphysical inquiry in philosophy of medicine, on the other hand, has focused primarily on the definitions of what counts as "health" versus what counts as "disease" (Engelhardt 1975; Boorse 2013). Yet both of these areas of inquiry in philosophy of medicine have left aside, for the most part, questions concerning the clinical process of medical diagnosis and the concepts that this process involves. There is a similar gap in the medical literature. Although diagnostics as well as heuristics and bias are extensively discussed in this literature, very little has been written on conceptual issues in the diagnostic process as a whole.

Given the importance of the diagnostic process in modern medicine, these gaps are both significant and surprising, especially because diagnosis is the starting point of the clinical encounter. In fact, before the treatment or prognostic evaluation of a patient can even begin, there must be at least a working diagnosis (and preferably an accurate one). Thus, a critical examination of the diagnostic process, and its prominent role in medical practice, seems to be well worth the effort. This book is meant to begin to address these gaps in the medical and philosophical literatures by engaging with some of the most important and overarching conceptual issues in the practice of clinical diagnosis.

Conceptual issues pertaining to diagnostic practice can be roughly divided into those that concern diagnostic *reasoning* and those that concern diagnostic *testing*. Both types of issues are discussed in this book. Furthermore, the methodology that you will find in what follows is an extension of the analytical methods of current philosophy of science and philosophy of medicine. These methods of analysis are not new, but what *is* new are the questions that I use these methods to address. These questions concern evidence, ethics, and justice as they relate to both diagnostic reasoning and diagnostic testing in the clinical setting.

My own reasons for studying and writing on the diagnostic process are not only academic but also personal. In my early twenties, I became seriously ill and was misdiagnosed, and therefore untreated, for many years. This experience was the cause not only of my genuine intellectual curiosity about diagnostic reasoning and testing in the clinical setting but also of my reasons for deeply caring about these things. It never hurts to remind ourselves that medicine is always about real people with real experiences, and we should therefore not only study it but also aim to improve it, in whatever ways we can.

I.2. BOOK ORGANIZATION AND CHAPTER THEMES

The book begins in Chapter 1 with a discussion of the dynamics of the patient–physician relationship, which is the foundation of the diagnostic process, and then moves to a discussion of the question of what counts as diagnostic evidence, as well as who gets to decide. The chapter introduces the interrelated themes of ethics and evidence as they pertain to clinical diagnosis, and these themes, the reader will notice, are continuously woven throughout the discussion in the rest of the book. In Chapter 2, the focus is on what needs to be taken into consideration when evaluating a diagnostic test in the clinical setting. In the chapter, I show that the evaluation of these components—accuracy, clinical effectiveness, and extraclinical value—requires not only scientific inquiry but also philosophical analysis. Accuracy is a minimum requirement that a diagnostic test must meet before we can ask the question of whether or not it is valuable to perform, but even once this is determined, other factors must also be taken into account as well. In particular, when evaluating a diagnostic test, we need to consider more than just a patient's measurable clinical outcomes. At least in some cases, the epistemic benefits of an accurate diagnostic test can make the results valuable for a patient, even when they do not directly influence that patient's treatment or prognostic outcomes. In Chapter

3, I discuss the process of diagnostic decision-making (DDM) in the clinical setting, via the evaluation of a specific example which is intended to show that, even in patient cases that might initially appear to be relatively uncomplicated, the process of DDM can be very complex and, in all instances, involves considerations of epistemology, ethics, and probability. Furthermore, the discussion in the chapter highlights the fact that the process of DDM is patient-specific and requires the evaluation of both qualitative and quantitative evidence, as well as a commitment, on the part of the physician, to shared decision-making with the patient. In Chapter 4, I use four case studies, three of which I observed while I was a visiting researcher at Columbia University Medical Center, to highlight and address issues pertaining to diagnostic uncertainty and its management. The cases I chose to examine in the chapter are what I consider to be "ordinary" or routine diagnostic cases, in terms of both the presenting symptoms and the inherent uncertainty in their differential diagnosis. Yet, as the discussion in the chapter shows, an effective management of diagnostic uncertainty must begin with an ability to recognize and acknowledge it in even routine cases in the clinical setting. However, even when diagnostic uncertainty is recognized, this alone is not enough for effective diagnostic practice: It must also be clearly communicated to the patient. In Chapter 5, I discuss the much talked about problem of overdiagnosis (which can in turn lead to potentially costly or harmful overtreatment) as well as the not much talked about problem of underdiagnosis (which can lead to repeated and unnecessary testing and clinic visits). In the chapter, I argue that looking to other forms of evidence, aside from that which comes from diagnostic testing, can help reduce the diagnostic uncertainty that in turn leads to these problems, by facilitating more accurate interpretations of tests conducted in the clinical setting. Finally, in Chapter 6, using the example of the coronavirus disease 2019 (COVID-19) pandemic, I explore the question of how to balance societal versus individual considerations when diagnostic tests are a scarce resource. As is well known, the purpose of diagnostic testing can be either for the promotion of public health or for the facilitation of the clinical care of individual patients. When diagnostic tests are scarce, we are sometimes forced to rank these, at times, competing purposes. I argue that when doing so, the primary responsibility of the treating physician is first and foremost to her individual patient rather than to the general public at large. For a medical researcher, on the other hand, the priority is reversed. However, because the practice of medicine always concerns the health of individuals, the goal is never knowledge acquisition alone, but instead always also its application.

One theme that I hope will emerge from the interrelated discussions in this book is that within the practice of clinical diagnosis, ethics and evidence cannot be separated, nor should they be. Because the goal of the diagnostic process is not just to acquire knowledge, but instead to also facilitate the health of actual people, it is an inherently ethical endeavor, and not just a scientific one.

Finally, I note from the start that the primary focus of my discussion in the chapters that follow is on questions of evidence, ethics, and justice as they relate to the clinical process of diagnosis. I leave aside the question of whether or not there is a "logic" of diagnosis and, if so, whether this logic resembles other types of scientific reasoning or is generalizable in some way [for a discussion of these issues, see Upshur (2005) and Sadegh-Zadeh (2011)]. I also leave open for others the metaphysical question of what kind of thing a diagnosis is [interested readers might find the discussion of psychiatric diagnoses in Sadler (2005), and Tekin (2016) to be helpful in this regard].

Chapter 1

Setting the Stage

1.1. THE PATIENT–PHYSICIAN RELATIONSHIP

The starting point of, and the foundation for, the process of clinical diagnosis is the relationship between the patient and the physician. Furthermore, the human-to-human interaction that occurs between a patient and their doctor is, in fact, also arguably the foundation for the entirety of modern medicine. This means that it is worth paying attention to! The relationship between the physician and the patient has both personal and scientific components, which are often intricately intertwined. This is one of the central themes of this book—that science and ethics, as discussed in much more detail in the chapters that follow, are inseparable in medical practice. Thus, in order to most effectively practice medicine generally, and diagnosis specifically, clinicians must at once be concerned with both scientific and ethical considerations.

As with most human relationships, the one between a patient and physician generally begins with an introduction, usually on the part of the physician. Even this simple interaction is important and should be approached thoughtfully. When introducing themself, the physician should state their name and role; using a title is not necessary. Instead, what *is* essential is that a professional, respectful relationship is established from the outset. Patients (unless they also happen to be physicians) are not trained in medicine and are therefore not "experts"[1] in the field. However, they are in fact equal partners in the patient–physician relationship, and this should be made clear by the physician from the start. Of course, the introduction is only the very beginning of the patient–physician relationship, and many have written extensively on the various ways in which the other aspects of this relationship should be conducted in practice (Emanuel and Emanuel 1992). Approximately 50–60 years ago, the dominant physician–patient relationship model was one of both epistemic and ethical paternalism. The doctor was the *pater*, whose role was to ensure that the patient received interventions that best promoted their health and well-being. Serving that end, the physician worked on their own, largely without patient input, to diagnose the patient and to choose an appropriate treatment or intervention (ethical paternalism), while presenting the patient only with carefully selected information along the way (epistemic paternalism[2]). The emphasis of this old-style model of doctoring was on the patient's health over and above everything else, including the patient's autonomy. But the problem with this model, as many have pointed out, is that physicians and their patients do not always share the same health goals. Determining what is the best decision in a given patient's case is not as simple as asking the question of "what is best" for the patient; it also requires asking the question of what the patient wants. And, in some cases, this is not

---

1. The definition of what counts as an "expert" is highly contested, and I leave aside the discussion of competing definitions here. Interested readers, however, are referred to Douglas (2008) and Watson (2020) for more details on this debate.
2. For further discussion of ethical paternalism, see Croce (2018).

the same thing as what the doctor wants. Because what the patient wants might differ from what the doctor wants, or what the doctor believes is best, it is now recognized that the patient should be able to have input into their diagnostic workup and ensuing treatment plan. This is because "" (Entwistle 2010, p. 1). It is from this nearly universal desire for self-rule that the concern for autonomy in patient–physician interactions arises. *Autonomy*, simply defined, is "self-governance" or the ability to make one's own decisions. Another way of stating this is that the term autonomy "typically designates an ability to . . . direct one's own choices and behaviors based on deliberation and reflection" (Racine et al. 2017, p. 8). In other words, in order for a decision to be considered autonomous, it must be made intentionally and with understanding and be made free from coercion or other controlling influences from the outside. Physicians should be aware that the way that they interact with their patients might either encourage or hinder patient autonomy. In addition to the influence of the physician, patients, like all people, are always located within a complex web of other interpersonal relationships, which can be very influential on their thought and decision-making processes. Some of these relationships support the patient's autonomy, and others undermine it. This means that determining what the patient wants and needs requires concerted effort on the part of the physician, which can be facilitated by carefully listening to the desires that the patient expresses[3] during the clinical encounter.

---

3. Of course, a patient's expressed interests might not necessarily coincide with their best interests. Nevertheless, respect for autonomous decisions, even if they are not the "best" decisions, all things considered, is nearly universally agreed to be preferable to paternalism, for reasons stated previously.

1.2. GATHERING EVIDENCE

In order to begin to help the patient, the physician will generally start with the goal of pursuing a diagnosis that explains the cause of the patient's condition. It is hoped that this diagnosis will, in turn, help facilitate an effective plan for treatment. Many clinicians consider a good (or "gold standard") diagnosis to be one that proposes a causal explanation, for two important reasons. First, knowing the cause of a patient's condition facilitates treatment (by allowing for the possibility of intervening on the cause); second, patients tend to both desire and respond positively to explanatory diagnoses rather than diagnostic labels that are not explanatory (Cournoyea and Kennedy 2014). Perhaps surprisingly, patients who understand *why* they have certain symptoms get better faster than patients who do not have this understanding (Van Ravenzwaaij et al. 2010), likely because understanding can give the patient hope, which we in turn know can significantly improve patient outcomes (Musschenga 2019). Thus, the clinical aim in the diagnostic process is usually to try to find a causal explanatory diagnosis for the patient's signs and symptoms.

In order to reach this goal of an accurate causal diagnosis, the physician needs to gather evidence. In evidence-based medicine (EBM), which is the currently accepted medical paradigm, the term *evidence* is a technical one. What EBM proposed when it was introduced in the 1990s was not that medicine should now begin to involve the use of "evidence" (the practice of medicine has always involved "evidence") but, rather, EBM proposed a new *hierarchy* of evidence (Evidence Based Medicine Working Group 1992):

> Evidence based medicine de-emphasizes intuition, unsystematic
> clinical experience, and pathophysiologic rationale as sufficient

grounds for clinical decision-making and stresses the examination of evidence from clinical research. EBM requires new skills of the physician, including efficient literature searching and the application of the formal rules of evidence.

At the top of this hierarchy are randomized controlled trials (RCTs) and meta-analyses, which are considered to be the strongest form of evidence, followed by observational studies, case studies, mechanistic reasoning, and, finally, at the bottom of the hierarchy, expert judgment or clinical expertise, which is considered to be the lowest form of medical evidence. The hierarchy of evidence is arranged in this way with the goal of minimizing bias, or systematic error, when gathering medical evidence, or pursing medical knowledge. The idea is that randomized, blinded trials are less amenable to bias from either allocation or expectation than are observational studies. Furthermore, it is thought that physician expertise might be especially prone to being clouded by biases of various sorts, including expectation biases and interpretation biases that might be based on incorrect or inadequate theories, and thus this form of evidence is ranked the very lowest on the pyramid. Overall, the main emphasis in the proposed method of EBM is on experimental data over and above theory. That is, although all data require interpretation, and therefore theory, at least at some level, when experiment and theory contradict one another, EBM tells us to rely on experiment (and revise the theory) rather than vice versa.

It is important to recognize that for the most part, EBM has focused on evidence for treatments and interventions rather than for diagnoses, about which it has (explicitly at least) relatively little to say. When tasked with evaluating a treatment or intervention, EBM advocates for physicians to look first at what the controlled studies state rather than at what experts recommend or their intuition suggests. In practice, this means that when an EBM practitioner or proponent uses the term evidence, they are almost always referring to an RCT and not to clinical experience, mechanistic reasoning, patient history, or anything else. However, this view of evidence is far narrower than what the method of EBM actually proposes. Furthermore, if this narrow view of evidence is too rigidly implemented in the clinical setting, it can be problematic with regard to patient care. In other words, if "evidence" just means "RCT," then there is no "evidence to suggest," for example, that penicillin is an effective treatment for streptococcus A, that the Heimlich maneuver prevents choking, or that the polio vaccine is effective. But of course we do, in fact, have evidence to suggest that these interventions are effective, and that is precisely because medical evidence is not, and should not be, limited to RCTs. As Braithwaite (2020) notes, "The fundamental problem with [the often-used EBM phrase] 'there is no evidence to suggest,' is that it is ambiguous while seeming precise" (p. 2149). Furthermore, he writes that this "mantra for EBM practitioners" can be harmful to clinical medicine because it can "signal to patients, physicians, and other stakeholders that they need to ignore intuition in favor of expertise, and to suppress their cumulative body of conscious experience and unconscious heuristics in favor of objective certainty" (p. 2149). The problem with this sort of method is that it ultimately inhibits shared decision-making and in that way is "corrosive to patient-centered care" (p. 2149).

Because clinical research alone, even in the best-case scenario, never settles health care decisions definitively (Goldenberg 2016), an appeal to a broader base of evidence (one that is not limited to statistical studies) seems to be not only justified but also necessary for effective clinical practice.

Furthermore, a view of medical evidence that excludes both physician and patient expertise and experience completely, whether intentionally or not, fails to recognize not only that important pieces of scientific evidence can be derived from these sources but also that ethical values are inextricably intertwined with every determination of what counts as evidence in any given situation, medical or otherwise. Once touted as the ideal, "value-free" science (and medicine) is now recognized by many as a state that is both unreachable and undesirable. Although those who once advocated for value-free science did so "because they understand values to be ideologically held and immune to rational evaluation" (Goldenberg 2013, p. 4), many now recognize that values can in fact be amenable to revision given empirical evidence and thus that they can be *good* reasons, not just reasons, upon which to base decisions. So although "there is no rule of logic that can help us decide whose interpretation of empirical experience is *the evidence*" (Shahar 1997, p. 114), this should not be a cause for despair. In medicine, individual values (on the part of both the patient and the physician) can and should matter in the determination of what counts as evidence.

However, a fundamental misunderstanding of what counts as medical evidence, as well as the role of values in determining this, is pervasive in clinical medicine today. Although foundational papers in the EBM movement (e.g., Sackett et al. 2000) explicitly state that decision-making under the paradigm of EBM should include information derived from experience and intuition, often this does not happen in practice. This is not only a problem with regard to making treatment decisions but also a problem in the diagnostic process because it is often assumed that only the results of diagnostic tests count as "real" evidence and that patient self-reports are unreliable, unhelpful, or even dispensable. However, this is far from being the case: In order to be an effective diagnostician, a physician must be

a pluralist about evidence. That is, the physician must learn to examine *all* of the available evidence, including the patient's report of
their own symptoms, not just the external evidence of patient signs,
such as those provided by diagnostic tests. In fact, qualitative evidence is so important in the diagnostic process that in 80 percent of
cases a correct diagnosis can be made on the basis of the patient history alone (Campbell and Lynn 1990). This is truly an astounding
statistic, if you take the time to think about it. What it means is that
even given all of our technological advances in recent years, the
single most effective way to improve diagnostic accuracy in the clinical setting is for the physician to learn how to listen—really listen—
to patients because they are the most important sources of reliable
diagnostic evidence. This, in turn, requires the use of metacognitive
skills, in order to arrive at this level of thoughtful diagnostic work,
and care in general.

The activity of listening to a patient, or "taking a patient history,"
is a skill that must be honed if one is to become an effective diagnostician. In the first instance, this skill involves learning to refrain from
cutting off the patient too quickly when the patient is telling their
story. Studies have shown that patients, when asked by a physician
to describe their concerns, are interrupted, on average, after only
18 seconds of talking (Beckman and Frankel 1984). This could be
due to the worry, on the part of the physician, that patients will go
on for too long if they are allowed to talk uninterrupted. However,
this concern seems to be unfounded: Marvel et al. (1999) found
that patients who were allowed to talk for as long as they needed
to, without interruption, spoke, on average, for only approximately
32 seconds—not really very long at all! By allowing the patient
to speak uninterrupted, you, the physician, are sending a signal to
the patient that you are listening, which sets the tone for a good
working relationship. In addition, it means that you probably *are*,

in fact, listening. If you listen to the patient, they will tell you what is wrong. That does not mean, of course, that the patient will know exactly what they have, how they got it, or how to treat it, but the patient does know *what is wrong*, and that is the information you must be able to home in on as a physician in order to reach an accurate diagnosis.

1.3. LISTENING TO THE PATIENT: EXAMPLE 1

Aside from cutting off the patient too quickly, another commonly made diagnostic mistake is to be dismissive of the patient's history and concerns (Kennedy 2013). There are many reasons why this sometimes happens during the diagnostic process. In some cases, it happens because the patient has a difficult-to-deal-with personality; in other cases, it happens because the patient's condition is complicated, rare, or otherwise difficult to diagnose. In cases such as these, it can be easy for the physician to blame the patient for their problems—to accuse the patient of hypochondria, malingering, attention-seeking, or self-sabotage. When a physician is not able to immediately diagnose the patient, the physician must be careful neither to place the blame on the patient nor to reach beyond the available evidence in attempting to make a diagnosis. Labeling a difficult patient as a "hypochondriac," for example, simply because the patient is difficult to interact with is not only rude but also a diagnostic mistake because the proper diagnosis of hypochondria requires the presence of clearly defined clinical findings associated with the condition, not simply that the physician cannot determine what is wrong or is tired of listening to the patient "complain." Instead of writing off a difficult-to-diagnose patient, physicians must instead be willing to listen carefully to their patients. After all, the patient is always the expert on their own symptoms. (This is the very definition of a "symptom" after all.) An example, as told to me by an internist in private practice, helps illustrate this point.

A 26-year-old woman with complaints of intermittent chest, abdominal, and leg pain came in to the office for routine care. She had a history of being born prematurely with gastroschisis, which was treated soon after birth. She also had a history of hysterectomy at age 23. Her cardiac evaluation (one month prior) was normal and she also had a negative stress test at that time. Her previous physician had labeled her as a "hypochondriac." However, an echocardiogram revealed coarctation of the aorta. The patient subsequently underwent vascular surgery to treat this condition and had resolution of all of her symptoms.

Aortic coarctation, or narrowing of the aorta, is generally, although not always, a congenital condition. However, in some cases, it is not detected until adulthood, depending on the severity of the narrowing. Symptoms of the condition include headaches, leg cramps, chest pain, and muscle weakness. Left untreated, the condition can lead to serious complications, such as brain aneurysm, aortic rupture, heart failure, or stroke. In this case, the patient's diagnosis was missed by the first physician because he essentially dismissed her concerns as "made up." Why this happened in this particular case is unclear; nevertheless, this example underscores the point that physicians must learn to listen carefully to their patients, in all cases, if they want to be effective diagnosticians. This does not mean, of course, that the physician needs to assume that the patient is correct in their interpretation of, or proposed causal explanations for, their symptoms. That is often (although not always) out of the realm of the patient's expertise.[4] However, if the physician is dismissive of the patient, the physician is less likely to listen to the patient and thus will be at risk of neglecting important pieces of evidence that come from the patient's self-report. This is problematic because neglecting evidence is always harmful to the diagnostic process. In other words, in order to be a good diagnostician, the physician needs to get the ethics of the physician–patient relationship correct. This is not simply because acting dismissively is both unkind and disrespectful; rather, it is because when a physician dismisses a patient's history, the physician also dismisses potentially vital pieces of evidence toward the diagnosis. Thus, best diagnostic practice requires a patient–physician relationship of mutual respect, even in cases in which a diagnosis cannot be made (immediately or at all).

One might object that not all patients are truthful and therefore that taking all patients at their word is not good for clinical diagnostic practice. It is true, of course, that some patients lie about or exaggerate their symptoms, but it is not the case that most of them do so. If you were to begin every patient interaction with an assumption that the patient is lying or exaggerating, there simply would be no possibility of practicing medicine effectively. And indeed, if a patient assumes you are not really listening to them, they will be more likely to overemphasize their symptoms in an effort to get the attention they need. Because of this, it is important to keep in mind that the starting point of the diagnostic process must begin with establishing a relationship of mutual trust: Both the patient and the physician must begin by taking each other at their word; there is no

---

4. Interestingly, some patients will themselves assume that they are hypochondriacs, or that their symptoms are psychological, when they are not. I personally observed one case in-clinic in which a Crohn's patient assumed that her steroid-induced retinopathy was "just stress" and another case in which a man believed that he was "just anxious" when he was in fact experiencing late-stage Grave's disease.

way for the relationship, or indeed the diagnostic process, to effectively proceed otherwise.

1.4. LISTENING TO THE PATIENT: EXAMPLE 2

As a second example of what can go wrong in the diagnostic process when a patient is treated dismissively, consider the following case study of a British surgeon in training (Wilson 1999):

> I had non-specific symptoms—malaise, fatigue—but with the photophobia, headache, and difficulty on my feet they were serious enough to warrant admission to the neurology ward for investigation. The investigations were thorough, but no cause was found.
>
> I was discharged back into the hands of a less than sympathetic university health service, and it was here that the mysterious spectrum of symptoms that graced my life earned me the title "malingerer," chiselled deeply into my notes and even deeper into the clinical opinions of all those who saw me thereafter.
>
> My aching joints were scrutinised by the rheumatologists. The neurologists put me under the inquisition again, trying to find some explanation for the interminable headache. Ultimately, as is often the case, I was directed to the psychiatrists. A label of "depression" was hung around my neck, and I spent several months at a loose end, my studies on ice, convinced that I was not psychiatrically unwell, yet being swayed increasingly to the point of view that I was somatising.
>
> A rather unhelpful faculty of medicine hindered my progress, and [a] constant headache was my shadow, my joints protested, and I had strange things happening to my skin—things I ascribed to a bad mattress, poor posture, worn out running shoes, and a hot bedroom rather than anything else.

In the end it was easier to live with the symptoms rather than be ridiculed [emphasis added] by those from whom I might seek advice. I learnt to accept the devastating effect that this malady was having on myself but most importantly on others. Constant pain, feeling permanently hung over, being unable to stand properly, and soaking erstwhile sleep partners, courtesy of night sweats, did not augur well for relationships.

It seemed odd to me that *the first time that a proper history was taken was when we knew the diagnosis* [emphasis added]. I had seen numerous specialists, but nobody had actually taken a full history; a point I had difficulty reconciling and even greater difficulty putting across. . . . When the serology came back I was delighted to find myself with Lyme disease. It was the greatest positive affirmation that I could have wished for. Soon after finals I underwent a rather unpleasant course of chemotherapy and then started in clinical practice. . . .

Regarding the effect my illness has had on my own clinical practice, I hope that I can reach the zenith of equanimity and openminded consultations that I might have benefited from. It was fortuitous to have discovered Lyme disease. I was not on any form of crusade.

Lyme disease is a multisystem inflammatory infectious disease that affects the skin, joints, heart, and nervous system. The etiologic agent of Lyme disease is the gram-negative spirochete *Borrelia burgdorferi*, which is transmitted mainly by tick bites. It is currently the most frequently recognized arthropod-borne infection of the central nervous system in both Europe and the United States (Mrazek and Bartunek 1999). Furthermore, according to the Centers for Disease Control and Prevention (2020), cases of

Lyme disease are both prevalent and significantly underreported. Complicating its diagnosis, the presentation of early Lyme disease is often nonspecific. Early symptoms of the infection often include fatigue, low-grade fever, generalized malaise, and arthralgia. However, because only approximately 50–60 percent of patients with Lyme disease recall a tick bite, and only 35–60 percent report the erythema chronicum migrans (bull's-eye) rash, early clinical diagnosis is often missed, causing the infection to become chronic or "late-stage." In late-stage Lyme disease, symptoms may include psychosis, anxiety, depression, mood swings, sleep disturbance, and attention-deficit/hyperactivity disorder. Presentation with these symptoms in the clinical setting frequently leads to the dismissal of the patient as a hypochondriac, as happened in the case study detailed previously. This is due, in part, to the fact that there is sharp disagreement over whether or not late-stage Lyme disease and its neuropathogenic effects even exist. For example, an opinion piece published in the *Polish Journal of Psychiatry* in 2010 stated that most purported cases of late-stage Lyme disease "can be described as induced hypochondria" and recommended that physicians not "forget the possibility of induced anxiety disorder or hypochondria" in patients who believe that "borreliosis is a chronic, serious disease" from which they suffer (Rorat et al. 2010).

The reasons for this disagreement over the nature of late-stage Lyme disease are, I believe, twofold. First, the treatment of Lyme disease for any length of time is expensive, and the treatment of late-stage Lyme is particularly expensive because it is often open-ended. Thus, the cost to either a private insurance company or a national health care system paying for such treatment is often substantial. Second, the controversy regarding late-stage Lyme disease is compounded by the fact that currently no test assay is available that can definitively determine whether or not active disease is present

(Stricker 2007). Because of this, the most recent clinical review in *BMJ* reports that the diagnosis of Lyme disease should be "mainly based on characteristic clinical signs and symptoms as interpreting the results of serological tests can be complex" (Kullberg et al. 2020, p. 369).

There are many interesting, and representative, components of the previous case study that are worth examining in further detail. The first one that immediately stands out is that although the patient in this case was White, male, well-educated, *and even a physician in training*, he was still treated dismissively by the doctors who saw him. This led to a delayed diagnosis, which caused the patient to suffer for many more years than he otherwise would have if he had not been treated this way. Although this sort of dismissal happens far more often to women, people of color, and those with a low level of education and/or socioeconomic status (Valles 2018; Yancy 2020), the fact that this happened to a patient who does not fall into any of these categories goes a long way toward demonstrating the pervasiveness of the problem of physicians acting dismissively toward their patients in the face of diagnostic uncertainty. It is normal for humans to feel uncomfortable in uncertain situations. And certainly no one—neither clinicians nor patients—likes medical uncertainty. Yet because, as discussed in further detail in the chapters that follow, medical uncertainty is always a part of clinical practice, physicians must learn to both acknowledge it and manage it, without blaming it on their patients. Learning to do this does not have to be overly complicated. In this particular case, the physicians could have started by simply taking a careful patient history instead of jumping directly to diagnostic tests, which in this case, as in many others, were not enough, on their own, to lead to an accurate diagnosis. Certainly, Lyme disease, given its notoriously nonspecific initial presentation, can be difficult to diagnose in its early stages.

There are many similar conditions. But a difficult-to-diagnose patient should not automatically be blamed for their illness, as this patient clearly was. Doing so is both a logical mistake and an ethical one. The logical error in this particular case was inferring from a lack of diagnostic evidence to a diagnosis of "malingering." That is, the treatment team in this case concluded that the patient was a hypochondriac because they were unable to find anything that they expected to find in their initial workup. This is a logical error in that the proper diagnosis of both physical and psychiatric illnesses (if they can in fact be separated—an interesting question that I do not address here) requires the presence of clearly defined signs and symptoms consistent with the diagnostic category, not simply a lack of expected findings. So, although it is not logically problematic for a physician to reason that "because I have not found any of the findings that one would expect to find with somatic diseases x, y, and z, therefore I can conclude that they are not the cause of the patient's illness," there is a problem in extending beyond this to the conclusion that therefore the patient's illness is "all in his head."[5]

The dismissal of the patient's history and concerns in this case was also an ethical error because it was disrespectful and left him feeling abandoned (because he was) by the medical profession, which in this case was also his own profession. This clearly caused added psychological anguish on top of the physical suffering for the patient. Although this particular case study ended well, with both an accurate diagnosis and an effective course of treatment, this was only because the patient eventually resorted to conducting his own research. What he discovered during his investigation prompted

---

5. Again, some patients will be convinced that their problems are psychiatric in nature when they are not. The point is that in order to help the patient, the physician must be both interested in and discerning regarding the details of the case rather than dismissive of them in any way.

him to request an antibody test for Lyme disease, which turned out to be positive. That is, the patient in this case essentially diagnosed himself. Not all patients are able to do this, of course, and even those who are able to are often denigrated for attempting to do so. But they should not be. Listening to a patient involves also listening to what the patient thinks might be the problem. As we have seen, this does not mean that physicians need to assume that patients are always correct in their attempts at self-diagnosis. However, it does involve recognizing that sometimes they are correct. What is ultimately important is not where the evidence toward an accurate diagnosis comes from but, rather, that a physician is willing to take into account all forms of diagnostic evidence, regardless of whether they are qualitative or quantitative in nature or whether they derive from patient- or physician-initiated investigation.

1.5. CONCLUSION

In this chapter, we have seen that the process of clinical diagnosis requires first establishing a therapeutic alliance between the patient and the physician and then drawing on, and evaluating, both qualitative and quantitative forms of evidence. Furthermore, as discussed in more detail in the following chapters, clinical diagnosis is also, in many ways, a very technical process that requires an understanding of scientific study design, probability theory, and statistical analysis. However, the discussion in this chapter was meant to show that the process of clinical diagnosis is not only *technical* but also *relational* because it starts with the relationship between the patient and the physician. Very often, getting to a correct diagnosis directly depends on the way in which the physician navigates this relationship: If a doctor is dismissive of a patient's concerns, the doctor risks cutting the patient off too quickly and possibly missing important pieces of evidence that could lead to a timely and accurate diagnosis. This means that doctors need to learn to carefully listen to their patients, not just because this is a nice, polite thing to do, in that it is respectful of the patient, but also because an accurate diagnosis depends on it—in more than 80 percent of cases. And, of course, in medical practice, accurate diagnoses are always the first goal because without them, both treatment plans and prognostic predictions are bound to fail.

Chapter 2

Testing

2.1. BACKGROUND

After taking a patient history, for simpler cases, a physician will perform a physical examination and then use pattern recognition, "based on the classification of disease and signs and symptoms" (Stanley and Campos 2013, p. 301), to make an immediate diagnosis, without having to use any diagnostic tests. Many dermatological conditions, for instance, are diagnosed in this way. In cases such as these, diagnostic testing is usually not required. But for the many types of cases that are not immediately recognized via pattern recognition, methods of probabilistic diagnostic reasoning must be used to diagnose the patient. In these cases, a physician will use the clinical assessment to generate a (usually informal) pretest probability of possible diseases, called the "differential," and then will select diagnostic tests to help rule in or out options within the differential. Because diagnostic testing is so often used in this process of generating a diagnosis, it is of pivotal importance for physicians to learn how to interpret these tests, and indeed to recognize that all tests always require interpretation. However, the question of how to evaluate and interpret a given diagnostic test is often not straightforward. Instead, it is one that requires both evidential and philosophical/conceptual analysis in order to answer.

In other words, the evaluation of a diagnostic test is both a medical process (Bossuyt, Lijmer, and Mol 2000; Bossuyt and McCaffery 2009; Brozek, Akl, and Jaeschke 2009; Rodger, Ramsay, and Fergusson 2012) and a philosophical one. Of particular importance in this process is the overarching question of what makes a diagnostic test worth performing in a given clinical situation. In other words, when evaluating a diagnostic test (or deciding whether or not to perform it), we want to know not only that the test is safe and accurate but also that it is either clinically effective or otherwise valuable. And the determination of whether or not a given diagnostic test reaches these standards in turn requires philosophical analysis.

To begin to see this, take the standard of diagnostic accuracy. Unless a diagnostic test is considered to be accurate, no physician or patient will be (or should be) interested in its results. So we can readily state, then, that accuracy is the minimum bar that all diagnostic tests must reach in order to merit further consideration. This minimum bar of test accuracy is determined via sensitivity (the true positive rate) and specificity (the true negative rate). These in turn can be determined either by observational study or by randomized controlled trial (RCT), and each of these methods has merits and pitfalls of its own. But in all cases, once a diagnostic test is determined to be accurate, our inquiry into its clinical value has only begun. That is, in general, a diagnostic test is not considered to be clinically valuable, or worth performing, unless it is not only accurate but also clinically effective. This means that unless performing a diagnostic test has a measurable net positive effect on a patient's clinical outcome, most physicians will not find reason to perform it. In order to determine, then, whether or not a given test is clinically effective, we must evaluate the effect (on a patient) of the test in question *plus* any resulting treatment or prevention strategies that might be administered to the patient based on the results of the test. There are some cases in which an accurate test might not be clinically effective but might be valuable in other ways that are not dependent on a patient's clinical outcome. In cases such as this, diagnostic tests can still be worth performing, as will be demonstrated by examples presented in this chapter, even when this will not directly affect the patient's treatment options or prognosis.

2.2. DIAGNOSTIC ACCURACY

As discussed previously, it is generally agreed upon that unless a diagnostic test is at least relatively accurate (no diagnostic test is 100 percent accurate), it will not be useful in clinical practice, and there is thus no point in performing it. This means that before we can determine whether or not a diagnostic test is effective in positively influencing a patient's clinical outcome, or is in some other way valuable, we must first determine whether or not it can be used to accurately diagnose the condition in question.

In order for this to be possible, the test must, in the first instance, be an accurate method of detecting or measuring a given object or quantity. But second, in order to have meaning in a medical context, the test must be given an interpretation. That is, what any given test result *means* is actually not a scientific question but instead a philosophical one. Thus, asking the question of whether or not a given diagnostic test is accurate is not exactly like asking whether or not a given tape measure is accurate. In the case of a tape measure, all we need to do is compare the tape measure with some reference standard, such as the standard meter in Paris, in order to determine whether or not it is accurate. But in order to determine whether or not a given diagnostic test yields accurate diagnoses, we need to compare the measurement capabilities of the test with that of a reference standard and to understand how to interpret the quantities that the test measures. For instance, in order to determine whether or not a given serum assay for cholesterol is accurate in diagnosing hypercholesterolemia, we need to know not only if the test accurately measures the amount of cholesterol in the blood but also whether or not to count whatever level it measures as "high," "low," or "normal." This means that we cannot escape philosophical analysis, even in the clinical process of differential diagnosis, precisely because even in a determination of diagnostic test accuracy, the *interpretation* of test results is required. This is so because without an interpretation, test results do not have any meaning, clinical or otherwise, for either the patient or the practitioner.

Of course, the determination of test accuracy is also a medical question and is one that has seen much recent discussion in the medical literature (Bossuyt et al. 2000; Bossuyt and McCaffery 2009; di Ruffano et al. 2017). Although RCTs have long been the evidence-based medicine (EBM) gold standard for determining both treatment and prevention efficacy, until more recently, they were not used to determine diagnostic test accuracy. The generally accepted line was, as Sackett wrote in 1996, p. 71, that "to find out about the accuracy of a diagnostic test, we need to find proper cross-sectional studies of patients clinically suspected of harbouring the relevant disorder, not a randomized trial." However, increasingly (Bossuyt et al. 2000; Bossuyt and McCaffery 2009; Rodger et al. 2012; di Ruffano et al. 2017), RCTs are now being used to determine diagnostic test accuracy and/or effectiveness for conditions ranging from diabetes to deep vein thrombosis (DVT). This method of determining diagnostic sensitivity and specificity raises some interesting philosophical questions.

To begin to evaluate the merits of determining diagnostic accuracy via RCTs, it is first helpful to remember that the main claim made by EBM proponents concerning RCTs is "that randomized trials provide better evidence than observational studies because the former allegedly rule out more confounding factors" (Howick 2011, p. 17). The principal epistemological reason for testing medical treatments and interventions with RCTs is that randomization supposedly mitigates selection and allocation biases. The worry is that without randomization, consciously or unconsciously, researchers might enroll subjects (or subjects might enroll themselves) in a particular experimental group, and such subjects might have an unknown property or confounding factor that modulates the treatment effect, thereby compromising the experiment. Randomization in clinical trials of treatment is meant to block this possibility. It is because of this that RCTs of therapeutic treatments and interventions, at least in the EBM literature, are considered to be stronger evidence for their effectiveness than observational studies. However, this claim has been sharply contested (Worrall 2007). One of the anti-randomization arguments that Worrall makes is that experimental groups can be made comparable by careful selection of control subjects, thereby making randomization unnecessary. This is undoubtedly also the case when conducting trials that assess the accuracy of diagnostic tests: Although it is certainly important to control for confounding factors in a trial of a diagnostic, this does not necessarily require that the trial be randomized with regard to subject selection.

It is also important to recognize that there are differences between RCTs that evaluate treatments and those that evaluate diagnostics. One difference is that it is very unlikely that a trial of the comparative effectiveness of a newer diagnostic test against an older diagnostic test could be influenced by a placebo or expectation effect, as is often the case in trials of treatments. It is also less likely that a trial of a diagnostic test would suffer from self-selection or allocation bias than would a trial of a therapeutic treatment or intervention, although it is certainly not impossible. For example, one might imagine a case in which one of the subjects in the study suspects that they might have the disease that the test being evaluated is designed to diagnose. This subject could potentially have reason to not want to have this disease diagnosed, perhaps for social or employment reasons, and therefore might have a preference to enroll in the group being given the test that the subject believes is less likely to pick up the disease. However, although a scenario such as this is certainly possible, it seems less likely to occur than selection bias in a trial of a therapeutic treatment or intervention. Thus, although subjects and researchers could potentially have some reason for wanting to have a positive (or a negative) result from a diagnostic test, and thus have a reason to prefer one test group over another, this scenario is less likely to occur than it does in trials of treatment therapies,[1] in which both the trial subjects and the researchers could quite easily have a preference for one group over another.

Aside from patient and researcher preferences, which seem less likely to introduce trial biases in the evaluation of the accuracy of diagnostic tests than in the evaluation of the efficacy of medical treatments, there is also the issue that, in certain instances, there can be population subgroup variations that affect the accuracy of particular diagnostics. This is one of the reasons that some EBM practitioners are calling for RCTs to be used to evaluate diagnostic test accuracy. If there can be properties of patients that modulate

---

1. Here, I am speaking only about trials of diagnostic accuracy. In trials of diagnostic accuracy plus treatment efficacy, selection and allocation biases would be just as common as in trials of treatment and occur for the same reasons.

the accuracy of certain diagnostic tests or procedures, the worry is that nonrandomized subject allocation in studies of their accuracy would imbalance the two test groups with respect to these properties and thus give unreliable data concerning the accuracy of the diagnostic being evaluated. However, again, these factors can, in most cases, be controlled for without the use of randomization, and indeed, the randomization of a finite population does not guarantee their even distribution.[2]

For example, one might be interested in evaluating whether a serum thyroid-stimulating hormone (TSH) level is more or less accurate in diagnosing hypothyroidism than a serum-free thyroxine (FT4) level compared with the clinical reference standard (gold standard) of TSH plus FT4[3] in patients who exhibit symptoms of possible hypothyroidism. TSH is a hormone produced by the pituitary, which stimulates the thyroid gland to release thyroid hormone into the bloodstream, whereas FT4 is a measure of the amount of unbound thyroid hormone circulating in the blood. Generally, an elevated TSH level is thought to indicate hypothyroidism, whereas a low level of FT4 indicates the condition. There are several patient factors that can affect each of these tests and that thus need to be controlled for when evaluating these diagnostics against one another. One of these factors is age: It is not uncommon for the TSH level to be elevated in the elderly even when hypothyroidism is not present (Bensenor et al. 2012). Another confounding factor is pituitary function. In those with abnormally low pituitary function,

---

2. To see this, imagine that I decided to divide my students into two groups in order to have an in-class debate. Using a random number generator to do this would not guarantee, for instance, that all of the A students, or all of the male students, etc. were evenly distributed between the two groups. Randomization guarantees perfect distribution only in infinite populations, and of course, RCTs, in actuality, never have infinite numbers of subjects.

3. For further discussion of this example and how it relates to the problems of over- and underdiagnosis, see Chapter 5.

TSH levels can be low or normal in the presence of hypothyroidism, rather than high. There are also factors that can affect testing of a FT4 level. Patients who are taking certain drugs (e.g., sulfa or aminoglycoside antibiotics, antihistamines, or lithium) can have low FT4 levels, even in the presence of normal thyroid function (Dong 2000).

Because of concerns about confounding patient factors that arise in cases such as this one, increasingly more often RCTs are being used to decide whether one diagnostic test is more accurate than another (compared with a reference standard). But as with RCTs of treatment therapies, it is not necessary that a trial be randomized in order to control for these factors. Careful distribution of patients into the two test groups (without randomization) can also mitigate confounding factors when they are known. Of course, not all confounding factors are known. Thus, the ideal way to control for this fact is to, when possible, give both tests to the same group of subjects. This is often not possible to do with treatment interventions (in some cases, it is impractical; in others, it is dangerous) but can be carried out in many cases in trials of diagnostic accuracy, as long as the two tests being compared are not too invasive or do not interfere with one another.

2.3. DIAGNOSTIC EFFECTIVENESS

Once the accuracy of a diagnostic test has been determined, and the test has been found to be a reliable way to diagnose the condition in question, then the effect of performing the test on clinical outcomes must be analyzed. As discussed previously, a clinically effective diagnostic test must not only be accurate but also, in some way, lead to a measurable improvement in the patient's health. Accuracy alone is not enough to determine clinical effectiveness because the information gained from diagnostic testing does not have a direct effect on patient outcomes[4]—only diagnostic, treatment, and preventative decisions made subsequent to obtaining test results are considered to have this kind of impact. And these decisions can only be made once the test has been given an interpretation that is medically relevant for the patient in question.

Thus, although the result of a diagnostic test is certainly important, we have to be concerned not only with the accuracy of the results but also with the interpretation of the results as well as with the question of whether or not performing the test will ultimately improve the health of actual patients, without a major risk of harm, in keeping with the overarching goal of medical practice. In order to determine this, we need to know whether or not a given diagnostic test is a good predictor not only of the condition it is intended to diagnose but also of treatment and/or prognostic outcomes for this condition. This information can, at least in theory, be determined via clinical trial evaluation. However, the best way to design a trial that reliably provides this information is not immediately straightforward. There are two reasons for this. First, there is the question of whether or not such a trial should be randomized, and second, there is the question of at what point in the trial the randomization or other form of control should take place, if it is employed. Proponents of RCTs for diagnostics (Rodger et al. 2012, p. 137) claim that

> while diagnostic cohort studies can inform us about the relative
> accuracy of an experimental diagnostic intervention compared

---

4. Although information from an accurate diagnostic test can have positive or negative indirect effects, see, for instance, (Cournoyea and Kennedy 2014).

with a reference standard, they do not inform us about whether
the differences in accuracy are clinically important, or the degree
of clinical importance (or the impact on patient outcomes)

and that, therefore, RCTs of diagnostic outcomes are needed
(Rodger et al. 2012). But although it is true that diagnostic cohort
studies that evaluate test accuracy do not tell us whether or not "the
differences in accuracy are clinically important"—that is, whether
or not they produce measurable effects in the patient—this, of
course, has nothing to do with the trial not being an RCT. Rather,
cohort studies of diagnostic accuracy are designed only to tell us
whether or not the test in question is accurate. If the study does this
by properly controlling for confounding factors, then it is no fault
of such a trial that it does not provide information about patient
outcomes—because this is not what it was designed to do. But eventually, we do want to have this information—that is, we do want to
know how a given diagnostic test will affect patient outcomes—and
so we do need to address the question of how to best design a trial
that provides this information.

In the first instance, a trial that will provide this information
must be a trial of diagnostic accuracy plus treatment efficacy because, as discussed previously, testing the accuracy of one diagnostic against the accuracy of another does not, in itself, constitute
a measure of the relative effect of the test on the clinical outcome of
a patient. Various ways have been suggested for designing trials that
will yield reliable information about the way that diagnostic tests
clinically affect patients. Generally, it is suggested that these trials
should compare "two diagnostic interventions (one standard and
one experimental) with identical therapeutic interventions based
on the results of the competing diagnostic interventions" (Rodger
et al. 2012, p. 137). This is because if both groups are given both

tests, and only those who test positive are given the treatment and those who test negative are not, then this would constitute a trial of only treatment and not test plus treatment, which is what is required when making a determination of the clinical effectiveness of a test. As a way around this, for example, one could compare treatment with L-thyroxine for hypothyroidism diagnosed based on an elevated serum TSH plus a low serum FT4 versus hypothyroidism diagnosed based only on a low serum FT4. One central concern in designing these kinds of trials is with the decision of where to put the points of control. Arguably, this ought to occur at two points: before the test being evaluated is performed (when subjects should be distributed to control for confounding factors that might affect the test result) and again after receiving the test result, when those who test positive for the condition in question should be distributed to control for factors that might affect the treatment being given. At the treatment point, double blinding should be used to mitigate confounding factors such as special treatment by investigators or an expectancy effect on the part of patients. In addition, at the treatment point, those who test positive should be divided into two groups, where one group is given the treatment in question and the other is given a placebo. Again considering our example of a trial that is designed to measure the relative clinical effectiveness of the diagnosis of hypothyroidism with serum TSH plus serum FT4 versus serum FT4 alone (and subsequent treatment with L-thyroxine), one would begin by distributing the subjects (to control for known confounding factors) into two groups, one that receives the TSH test and the FT4 test and one that receives the FT4 test. Then, those who test positive in each group would be given either L-thyroxine or a placebo, and then each of the groups would be followed and evaluated for measurable clinical outcomes, such as a change in symptoms and/or serology.

2.4. EXTRACLINICAL VALUE

A further question to consider when evaluating a diagnostic test is whether or not an accurate test can be considered to be valuable even when it has no measurable effect on a patient's clinical outcome and thus would not in any way change what a physician would (or could) do for the patient. In other words, it is important to ask the question of whether or not a diagnostic test that has no clinical effectiveness can yet have some other kind of value and thus be worth performing.

For example, one might ask whether an accurate diagnostic test for an untreatable, unpreventable disease is valuable or worth performing. If the disease is not treatable or preventable, then testing for it will not change a patient's clinical outcome in any way, and thus the test, by definition, would not be clinically effective. However, the question of whether or not tests such as this can have some other sort of medical value is currently being debated. On the one hand, some have argued that "test selection should be restricted to those diagnostic tests whose results could change the physician's mind as to what should be done for a patient" (Sox et al. 2007, p. 5). If this is the criterion for diagnostic value, then no clinically ineffective tests could ever be considered to be valuable or worth performing. On the other hand, some research suggests that many patients want to know what is wrong with them, even when a treatment for their illness or condition is not available (Lijmer and Bossuyt 2009). And thus physicians are divided over whether an accurate test for an untreatable disease should ever be performed. A careful answer to the question of whether or not clinically ineffective tests can yet have some sort of value requires an examination of value in the medical context more generally. If we analyze value as inextricably tied to patient outcomes, then a diagnostic test will only be valuable if it is effective. On the other hand, if we admit the presence of value that is not directly tied to measurable clinical outcomes, then a test that provides a patient and a physician with an accurate diagnosis can be considered valuable even when it does not directly improve the patient's health.

For example, in some cases, a diagnosis can itself be a therapeutic tool and bring epistemic benefits to a patient and physician by allowing them to understand or make sense of the condition even when the clinical outcome remains unchanged. Diagnoses can do this even in cases in which they are incomplete or only partially correct by making the disease intelligible to the patient and the health care provider, even when they do not allow the physician to develop any treatment or outline any specific prognosis. These benefits then are separate from the therapeutic benefits of any medical treatment developed from such a diagnostic explanation. In other words, the understanding derived from an explanatory diagnosis is therapeutic to patients, and sometimes to the physician, in its own right. That a diagnosis can be a therapeutic tool speaks to the value of understanding in the clinical setting and the importance of pursuing diagnoses even in cases in which they will not lead to further action (Cournoyea and Kennedy 2014). This means that epistemic benefits can make an accurate diagnostic valuable even when that diagnostic is not clinically effective.

However, others (e.g., Lijmer and Bossuyt 2009) have explicitly argued against this view. Their claim is that what makes a diagnostic test valuable for the patient and/or the physician is not its degree of correspondence with the truth but, rather, whether or not that diagnosis, and the subsequent treatment for the condition, will save the patient from future physical or mental suffering. For an untreatable, unpreventable disease, this would not be the case because an accurate diagnosis would not prevent future disease progression. This kind of view, which equates the value of a diagnostic test solely with its ability to prevent patient suffering, would render the diagnosis of an untreatable, unpreventable disease as having no medical value. However, this position completely ignores the fact that many patients and physicians really do want to know what is wrong with the patient, even when nothing can be done about it.

Consider, for instance, the question of whether or not a diagnostic genetic test for Huntington's disease can be considered to be medically valuable. There are two possible situations in which to consider the value of such a test. The first is a situation in which a patient is exhibiting symptoms that could possibly be due to Huntington's disease (and thus not treatable) or could possibly be due to something else that is treatable. In this situation, the physician might run the test for Huntington's disease in order to rule out that condition while simultaneously searching for a treatable cause of the patient's symptoms. In this case, the diagnostic test could be considered to be clinically effective if it eventually facilitated the diagnosis and subsequent treatment of the patient's condition. The second case to consider is that of giving the test to a healthy person, perhaps with a family history of the disease, so that person could know whether or not they will develop the disease in the future—and perhaps, in this way, relieve the mental suffering that many patients experience due to medical uncertainty. In this case, because there is currently no available treatment for Huntington's disease, the test cannot be said to be clinically effective. However, it still seems reasonable to say that the test has some kind of value, precisely because the patient has a desire to know their health prognosis. If knowing that they will develop Huntington's disease in the future (or not) is beneficial to the patient, for epistemic or other reasons, then performing the test seems to have medical (if not directly measurable) value.

The main argument that is often advanced against this kind of view of medical value is that because medicine is an applied practice that aims at improving patient health, it would be a waste of both time and monetary resources to perform a test that will not in any way improve the measurable health outcomes of the patient (Coon et al. 2014). But something about this view of medical value, although it is admittedly difficult to articulate, seems to be too narrow. Although it might not always be in the best interest of society to diagnose people with untreatable diseases (or, alternatively, to diagnose them with conditions that do not cause any negative symptoms[5]), and this is certainly something that should be taken into account in clinical practice generally, this does not mean that performing a clinically ineffective diagnostic test is never in the best interest of a particular patient. In some cases, there really does seem to be value in an accurate medical diagnosis even when there is no direct clinical benefit from that diagnosis. That is, even when nothing in terms of treatment or prevention can be done for a patient, an accurate medical diagnosis could (very reasonably) be of value to both the patient and the physician.

In contrast to this line of argument, Hofmann (2016) explicates a different view of what it means for a diagnostic test to be valuable. He begins by drawing a distinction between "knowledge" (which he defines as "information about a potential health condition following from an accurate or actionable test", p. 13) and "risk information" while leaving open any precise definition of "knowledge," "information," or "accurate." What seems to be important for his view is that the results of a diagnostic test do not count as knowledge (and thus

---

5. Accurately diagnosing a condition that does not negatively affect a patient in any way (in either the short or the long term) is considered to be "overdiagnosis," which is a topic that is discussed in more detail in Chapter 5.

are not valuable) if either (1) the test is inaccurate or (2) the test is accurate but "unactionable." Certainly in no case should we be concerned with inaccurate tests or their results. Instead, test accuracy is definitely a minimum bar that must be met before we can even begin to think about whether or not a given diagnostic test is worth performing. In other words, Hoffman is correct in arguing that if some piece of medical information is inaccurate, then there is no reason to care about it at all. But where his view goes astray is when he argues that any medical information that is unactionable is therefore also not valuable. Based on the previous discussion, there seem to be cases of genuine diagnostic value even when the results of a given diagnostic test do not lead to measurably improved clinical outcomes for the patient in question. But according to Hofmann, the only thing that we ought to care about is whether or not the test results will make any improvement in a patient's health. He writes that if the result of a test is accurate but "nothing can be done to improve . . . health, there appears not to be any compelling reason" to perform the test (p. 13). This view is directly opposed to the one I am proposing here, so let me try to make clearer the reasons I oppose it.

2.5. EXAMPLE: EFFORT THROMBOSIS

Consider the following case study:

> A 42-year-old woman presented in the emergency department with a severely swollen left arm. She stated that when she had gone to bed the night before there was no swelling in that arm, but that when she woke up seven hours later the left arm was approximately twice the

size of the right. The attending physician suggested that perhaps the patient had "slept wrong."

After a shift change, a second attending physician examined the woman and took a more careful patient history. There was a history of a peripherally inserted central catheter line that was in place for eight months, fourteen years prior, for the intravenous treatment of a bacterial infection. This physician ordered a duplex ultrasound, which revealed two DVTs—one in the subclavian vein and another in the distal axillary vein. The subclavian vein thrombosis had completely occluded that vessel and was thereby determined to be the cause of the left arm edema. The patient was then questioned about her activity in the days leading up to the DVT. She stated that she had been lifting weights and swimming in the days before. These activities were a usual part of her exercise routine. The attending physician decided to discharge the woman on oral anticoagulation and instructed her to follow up with a vascular surgeon the following day. He explained to her the risk of pulmonary embolism, which could happen if the blood clot traveled to one of the lungs, and told her that her arm would likely remain swollen for several years.

After discharge, the woman consulted with a vascular surgeon as instructed. The surgeon suspected what is known as "effort thrombosis," secondary to venous thoracic outlet syndrome (VTOS), and told the woman that she would need immediate surgery to remove the clot or else she would risk losing function in her arm permanently. The woman underwent thrombolysis three days later. During the procedure, the preliminary diagnosis of VTOS was confirmed via venogram, and the woman was referred to a large university hospital for first rib resection and scalenectomy, which took place twelve days later.

Unlike DVT of the lower extremities, which is most often caused by inactivity, subclavian vein thrombosis is usually caused by vigorous activity or extensive use of the upper extremity. This kind of "effort" thrombosis of the axillary subclavian vein usually occurs in patients with excessive arm activity in the presence of one or more compressive elements in the thoracic outlet (Urschel and Patel 2008). Furthermore, the condition occurs most commonly in young, healthy male athletes in their twenties and thirties who use "arm over the head" motions repeatedly in their sport. The condition occurs with the highest frequency in swimmers, but it has also been diagnosed in hockey players, climbers, baseball players, gymnasts, dancers, and water polo players. It occurs when the scalene muscles, which are engaged when the arm is raised above the head, become overdeveloped, pull up on the first rib to which they are attached, and thereby compress the space between the clavicle and the first rib, which is known as the "thoracic outlet." When this space becomes narrowed over time, the subclavian vein, which runs through it, can become pinched and scarred. This pinching and scarring slows the flow of blood through the vein, which increases the risk of developing a clot. However, because the pinching is painless, the patient is not aware of it until a clot forms and thereby partially or completely occludes the subclavian vein, causing significant edema in the arm. Clots generally form after a period of intense activity and may take place years after the compression first begins.

Fifty to sixty years ago, treatment for this condition was conservative and involved oral anticoagulation, elevation of the arm, and activity restriction. Chronic disability was also common (estimates put it at upwards of 80 percent). More recent guidelines suggest immediate clot removal (thrombolysis) followed by the removal of the first rib and anterior and middle scalene muscles to create space in the thoracic outlet to allow the subclavian to "pop" back open or, when this does not happen, for collateral vessels to have room to develop and redirect blood flow from the arm back to the heart. Success rates (defined as full use of the arm and minimal swelling without the need for long-term anticoagulation) post surgery are estimated at 85 to 90 percent (Alla et al. 2010).

2.6. ANALYSIS

> After undergoing first rib resection surgery, the patient was subsequently placed on a subcutaneous anticoagulant medication (which is standard protocol after this procedure). Two days after the surgery, the attending hematologist and his residents visited the patient in the hospital on their rounds. The patient inquired into when she should be tested for clotting disorders. The attending turned to his residents and said, "Never. There is a structural reason for the thrombosis. If we tested for clotting disorders we would simply be looking for a reason to put her on lifelong anticoagulation."

The hematologist's answer in this case is interesting given that the literature is divided on the question of whether or not to test for hypercoagulability in cases of thrombosis due to VTOS. Some authors argue that such testing is necessary only when patients present with an upper extremity DVT that is not associated with activity (Likes et al. 2013), whereas others have found that as many as 50 percent of patients with effort thrombosis due to VTOS also have associated thrombophilia (Washington University St. Louis, https://tos.wustl.edu/). Still others have argued that even if a patient is found to have a thrombophilia, treatment is not necessary if there is an underlying structural cause for the blood clot. The idea behind this recommendation seems to be that only the primary cause of the VTOS needs to be addressed and secondary or tertiary causes can safely be ignored. The hematologist in this case, if he was aware of this literature, likely reasoned that the chance of a reoccurrence of an upper extremity DVT would be very low even if the woman turned out to have a thrombophilia, and thus that the results of such testing would essentially not be actionable from his point of view—that is, they would not change in any way what he would or could do for the patient. However, because the woman *wanted* to know whether or not she had a clotting disorder, she asked her primary care physician to run a thrombophilia panel a few months later. It turned out that she was heterozygous for a prothrombin II mutation. She then took this information to a second hematologist in order to determine whether or not this finding warranted lifelong anticoagulation. It was ultimately determined, via an extensive discussion in the clinic, that it did not. However, the woman expressed that she was glad to know about this clotting disorder because she would now take precautions when flying, choosing a birth control method, etc. that she would not have known to do had she not been tested for thrombophilia.

In this case, then, we might say that the results of this test for a prothrombin II mutation were not actionable from the hematologist's point of view (in terms of prescribing lifelong anticoagulation), even though they were actionable from the patient's point of view (in terms of lifestyle changes). For Hofmann, it might be the case that this information counted as "valuable" for this patient. But this case then raises the question of whether there ever is a truly unactionable diagnostic test. Even in the case of an untreatable, unpreventable disease such as Huntington's disease, it is difficult to say that any test result (whether positive or negative) is completely unactionable. It might, at the very least, be actionable in terms of a patient's life plans or lifestyle, and if this is true, then it means that the value of a diagnostic test, even on Hofmann's view, is not limited to measurable improved clinical outcomes for the patient.

2.7. CONCLUSION

As the discussion in this chapter is meant to show, when evaluating a diagnostic test, we need to consider, in addition to safety, three components: accuracy, clinical effectiveness, and extraclinical value. Doing this requires not only scientific inquiry but also philosophical analysis. As we have seen, accuracy is a minimum requirement that a diagnostic test must meet before we can ask the question of whether or not it is valuable to perform. Accuracy is best determined via a clinical trial that carefully controls for confounding factors. Ideally, this should be performed by comparing the results of a new test and an existing test against a reference standard, all performed on the same group of patients. When this is not possible, the next best trial design is to distribute the trial subjects in such a way that there is an even allocation of all known relevant subgroup variations. This, as in clinical trials of treatment therapies, does not require randomization. The clinical effectiveness of a diagnostic test, on the other hand, must be determined by evaluating the test plus any subsequent treatment and/or prevention measures. A trial that evaluates diagnostic test effectiveness should be controlled at two points: prior to the test being administered and prior to the treatment being given. Although controlling for confounding factors such as subgroup variation and bias in trials of test effectiveness is important, this does not necessarily require that the trial be randomized.

Finally, when evaluating the clinical value of a diagnostic test, we should consider more than just a patient's measurable clinical outcome. At least in some cases, the epistemic benefits of an accurate diagnostic test can make it valuable for a patient—perhaps by alleviating the suffering that can be caused by medical uncertainty—and thus worth performing, even when it does not directly influence that patient's treatment or prognostic outcomes. Furthermore, even tests that do not improve measurable outcomes in a patient might, at the very least, be actionable in terms of life plans or lifestyle, and if this is true, then it means that the value of a diagnostic test is not limited to measurable improved clinical outcomes for the patient. Thus, an examination of the issues that arise with questions of how to evaluate diagnostic tests is extremely important for clinical medical practice. We need to know not only that a test is accurate but also for what purpose we are testing, because the value of a diagnostic test is not limited to its clinical effectiveness.

Chapter 3

Decision-Making

3.1. BACKGROUND

In the previous chapter, we discussed conceptual issues in the interpretation of diagnostic tests, as well as some of the reasons for performing diagnostic evaluations that go beyond their clinical effectiveness. The interpretation of diagnostic tests is, however, part of a broader activity in clinical practice, which is a process commonly referred to as diagnostic decision-making (DDM). In this chapter, I use this term to encompass the entire process of clinical and evidential reasoning that is used to make estimations of, and decisions regarding, patient diagnosis.

Although, as discussed in this chapter, this process is often multifaceted and complex, it is nevertheless used throughout clinical practice from the most routine cases to the most difficult ones. Because all physicians engage, either formally or informally, in the process of DDM, it is vitally important to understand how the process works (actually), as well as how it should work (ideally).

3.2. THE PROCESS OF DIAGNOSTIC DECISION-MAKING

The process of DDM involves the consideration of how to understand and characterize information gained from the medical history and physical examination, as well as decisions regarding whether and which diagnostic tests and procedures should be used when considering the possible causes of a patient's problem and, finally, how to best interpret these tests. As discussed in Chapter 2, in some instances, a physician might make a diagnosis and suggest treatment based on the interview and examination alone, whereas in many others, diagnostic tests or procedures may be required during the process of differential diagnosis, which is the probabilistic method of diagnostic reasoning used to rule in or rule out diagnostic options. Thus, DDM brings together both the logical and the evidential components of the diagnostic process.

As discussed in Chapter 2, when considering whether or not to perform diagnostic testing, the first concern is always with the accuracy of the test or procedure. Accuracy, recall, is a function of the specificity (how well the test excludes patients without the disease) and sensitivity (how well the test identifies patients with the disease) of the diagnostic. Once a diagnostic test is found to be accurate—that is, once it is found to provide reliable epistemic information about the patient's condition—the question of whether or not it is worth performing remains. As noted in Chapter 2, the most generally accepted position in current medical practice is that unless performing a test will lead, via treatment or lifestyle intervention, to an improved (and measurable) patient outcome, it should not be performed. However, the information provided by diagnostic testing does not, on its own, have a direct effect on a patient's outcomes; rather, it is what we *do* with this information that has an impact (positive or negative) upon the patient's health. Thus, in order to determine whether or not performing a test will in turn lead to improved patient health, one needs to know whether a given diagnostic test is a good predictor not only of the condition it is intended to diagnose but also of treatment outcomes for this condition. This consideration too must enter into the DDM process: One might decide to perform a test only if it has been shown to not only accurately diagnose a given condition but also lead to improved patient health in those with the condition it diagnoses.

Once a patient's condition has been diagnosed, medical decisions regarding treatment must then be made. Treatment decisions can be quite complex and involve evaluating (generally on the basis of data from randomized controlled trials or observational studies) whether or not a treatment is therapeutically effective, whether or not it is affordable, whether or not it will interact with other patient treatments and/or comorbid conditions, and whether or not the long-term benefits and/or effects of the treatment are in line with patient expectations and values. Furthermore, in some cases, it might be important to take into consideration *how* a therapy or intervention works, in order to gain adequate informed consent.[1]

Because this book focuses primarily on the diagnostic process rather than on treatment considerations, for the most part I do not discuss those issues in detail here. However, some treatment considerations do factor into the diagnostic reasoning process, for a

---

1. This is sometimes the case when ethical considerations impact treatment decisions. For example, if the proposed mechanism of a given treatment would conflict with a patient's moral values, then the patient should be made aware of this. For a more complete discussion of the connection between mechanisms of action and informed consent, see Kennedy and Malanowski (2018).

variety of reasons—including ethical, financial, and practical ones. This means that deciding whether or not to pursue a diagnosis can potentially have ramifications in all of these areas. Furthermore, multiple decisions often need to be made regarding diagnosis in each patient case. In order to facilitate these decisions, DDM, practiced well, should draw on insights from decision science, economics, probability theory, and theoretical models of the physician–patient relationship and shared decision-making. Thus, DDM incorporates both quantitative approaches, such as using Bayes' theorem to determine pre- and post-test probabilities, and qualitative approaches, such as discussing with patients their values when estimating the expected utility of a given diagnostic test. In addition, the process of DDM involves both the concerns of the physician (e.g., the harms vs. benefits of a test or an intervention) and those of the patient (e.g., how the patient feels about these harms or benefits). As such, DDM is a science that can be understood only from a multidisciplinary perspective.

3.3. EXAMPLE: RECURRENT SINUSITIS

In order to better understand both the process of DDM in clinical practice and the philosophical issues that this process raises, it is helpful to look at an example. Consider the following fictional but plausible scenario:

> A 32-year-old male presents to the ear, nose, and throat clinic with facial pain, fatigue, low-grade fever, and a history of chronic/recurrent sinusitis. Furthermore, he reports that he experiences six to ten such infections per year and has so continuously for the past five or six years. These infections have been diagnosed via computerized

tomography (CT) scan and treated by his primary care physician with ten to fourteen days of antibiotic therapy each time. The infections resolve successfully (temporarily), only to return after a few weeks or months. The patient has also undergone allergy testing, with no significant environmental allergies documented. The patient is frustrated and expresses a desire to find the "cause" of his ailment so that the recurrences of sinusitis can be stopped.

In this case, the clinical encounter will begin, as most do, with a medical interview in order to gather evidence toward making a diagnosis of the cause of the patient's recurrent illness. The questions asked of a patient during this interview will differ depending on the presentation and the specific patient circumstances. In some cases, such as in the emergency setting, there will be little time for questioning at all, and the physician will proceed directly to physical examination. In this example, however, the situation is not emergent. Instead, the pressing matter is to determine why the patient's infections are recurring so that they can be stopped. If the physician in this case works under the assumption that the patient's infections were properly diagnosed and did in fact respond to antibiotic therapy, then the physician would next need to perform a physical examination to determine if further diagnostically relevant information can be obtained. However, with sinusitis, as with many conditions, the condition cannot be diagnosed on the basis of the examination alone. A patient who presents with recurrent nasal swelling, sore throat, fatigue, and lymphadenopathy, for example, could be suffering from a number of illnesses, including viral upper respiratory tract infection, allergies, or bacterial sinusitis. However, a patient who has a history of documented bacterial sinusitis, and does not have environmental allergies, is more likely to be experiencing a recurrence of this condition rather than a viral infection. Absent the history of bacterial sinusitis, the opposite would be true (a viral infection would be more likely). Thus, in this instance, as in many others, the diagnostician must use the information gathered from the patient history in conjunction with clinical data because the clinical data alone would not be enough to ensure accuracy in diagnosis.

In this particular example, the physician, based on patient history and a physical examination, could reasonably rule out causes for the patient's condition other than recurrent bacterial sinusitis and then diagnose the patient with this condition. Once the patient has been diagnosed with recurrent bacterial sinusitis, the physician will not only need to treat the current infection but also need to investigate the underlying cause of the recurrent infections, with the goal of making a causal diagnosis that will facilitate resolution of these infections.

3.4. CAUSAL DIAGNOSES

Causal diagnoses (as opposed to label or syndromic diagnoses), particularly those that posit pathophysiological mechanisms, are generally considered to be the gold standard for medical diagnosis (Smith and Francesca 2007) because it is thought that understanding the underlying pathophysiology of an illness best allows for effective treatment. Causal diagnoses are not always possible to obtain, nor are they generally singular,[2] but when they are obtainable, they are

---

2. Causal explanations in medicine are often complex and multifactoral. This has implications for both clinical medicine and public policy. For example, in the state of South Carolina, death certificates must indicate the primary cause of death as well as secondary and tertiary causes. For example, cause of death might be listed as "cardiac arrhythmia as a result of severe hyponatremia, due to SIADH."

almost universally considered to be preferable to diagnoses that do not describe the cause of the illness (Knotternus and Buntinx 2008). In this particular case, uncovering the underlying reason for the recurrent bacterial sinus infections is important because unless the cause of the issue is identified and treated, the infections will most likely continue to recur.

In order to try to find the underlying pathophysiological cause of a patient's complaint, the physician will often begin by making a differential list of the most likely predisposing conditions. For chronic or recurrent sinusitis, these include

- allergic reactions (which cause the nasal passages to swell);
- nasal passage abnormalities such as nasal polyps or a deviated septum;
- an immune system disorder (either acquired or primary); and
- asthma.

Although there are certainly other possible underlying conditions that present with these signs and symptoms, the initial differential list is composed of only the most likely ones. If all of the conditions in the differential are eventually ruled out, then the physician will create a new differential that includes other, less likely, conditions.

In order to eliminate conditions in the differential and eventually arrive at an accurate diagnosis, the physician needs to evaluate, either formally or informally, the probability of each of the conditions individually. This is generally done via an appeal both to personal experience and to published data. Even in the era of evidence-based medicine, clinical experience provides a wealth of knowledge that can assist in making an accurate diagnosis. Published data can also of course provide diagnostic evidence. However, although both sources of evidence are important, both are subject to biases. In the former, biases include physician overconfidence (which can lead to disinterest in investigating supplemental decision support); a tendency to assume that the current patient has a condition that the physician has previously seen; and premature closure, which is the narrowing of diagnostic options too early in the process of differential diagnosis so that the correct diagnosis is never seriously considered (Berner and Graber 2008). In the latter case, the biases most often result from faulty clinical trial design (Emmanuel, Wendler, and Grady 2000) or from an assumption that the available trial data are applicable to a particular patient when they are not.

Furthermore, there is often disagreement among physicians about the relative probabilities of the conditions in the same differential. This disagreement is due both to differing clinical experiences and to the fact that different physicians read different journals. For instance, primary care physicians are more likely to read articles in primary care journals, which report the prevalence of disease in unselected patients, whereas specialists more often read journals that report studies of patients who have been referred to specialists. Understanding the prevalence of each of the conditions in the differential is thus pivotal in facilitating a correct and timely diagnosis.

Once probabilities (either formally or informally) have been assigned to the various conditions in the differential, the physician must then decide what, if any, diagnostic testing to perform in order to decide between them. Of the conditions on the list in our example, allergies and structural abnormalities are far more common than primary immunodeficiency diseases. As such, they should be investigated first and, in this case, can be ruled out on the basis of previous allergy testing and CT scan evaluation, respectively. Asthma, which is also more common in the general population than immunodeficiency disease, can in turn be ruled out via a careful patient history and/or simple testing. This leaves only immunodeficiency disease in the differential. Although it is the last remaining possibility in the initial differential, this does not mean that the patient definitely has such a condition, but it does raise the probability that he does, especially given the frequency of bacterial infection reported (which would be uncommon in someone with a well-functioning immune system).

At this point in the diagnostic process, the physician would likely form a new differential that includes both HIV/AIDS (the most common form of secondary immunodeficiency) and common variable immune deficiency (the most common form of primary immune deficiency). Given this new differential, the physician would then proceed to diagnostic testing in order to gather further evidence toward a diagnosis.[3]

3.5. PROBABILITIES

Because the physician in this case suspects an immune disorder, they will want to use diagnostic testing to determine the likelihood that the patient has one of these conditions. Importantly, this likelihood, or probability estimate, depends on both the pre- and post-test probability that the patient has the disease in question. The pretest probability of a disease is the probability that disease is present before any testing is conducted. This probability will depend on whether or not, given the patient history, the patient is in a high- or low-risk group for the condition in question. The post-test probability of a disease depends on the pretest probability as well

---

3. In an acute setting, such as the emergency department, diagnostic testing would more likely be performed all at once instead of sequentially, depending on the acuity of the presenting problem.

as the accuracy (sensitivity and specificity) of the test that is being performed. Thus, there is no such thing as being absolutely certain of what a test result means; it varies from one patient to another depending on the patient's pretest probability. Having a positive test result does not necessarily mean that a patient has the condition, nor does having a negative test result mean that the patient does not have the condition. However, clearly, these results do affect the likelihood of whether or not the patient has the condition that the test is intended to diagnose.

Suppose that the patient in our example is in a low-risk group for secondary immunodeficiency due to infection with the HIV virus and is also seronegative for the virus. In that case, the physician can reliably remove this condition from the differential list. Of course, as noted previously, even with a negative test, one cannot be certain that the patient is not infected with HIV, but when the pretest probability of the condition is low, and the test is negative, the likelihood of the patient having the disease is very low.

Once secondary immune deficiency has been ruled out, the possibility of a primary immunodeficiency in a patient who has frequently recurring infections of the skin or respiratory tract should be investigated. More than 200 primary immunodeficiency diseases are recognized by the World Health Organization. Common variable immune deficiency (CVID), so named because it is the most common one (but still very rare; according to the National Institutes of Health, the incidence in the population is approximately 1 in 25,000 to 1 in 50,000 people worldwide, although the prevalence can vary across different populations), can be tested for with simple and relatively inexpensive serum tests because it is characterized by low levels of serum immunoglobulins. The low level of these antibodies in CVID is the underlying cause of the increased susceptibility to infection in patients with the condition.

Furthermore, patients with CVID also have an increased incidence of autoimmune or inflammatory manifestations and susceptibility to cancer compared to the general population. The diagnosis of CVID is usually made in the third or fourth decade of life, so this condition should be suspected in patients of this age who present with any of the previously mentioned conditions.

In our particular example, the patient has at least two markers that increase the pretest probability that he has this condition: frequent respiratory infections (Wood et al. 2007) and age in the mid-thirties. Thus, diagnostic testing for CVID, given the previously mentioned markers, seems reasonable in this specific case, particularly because it is minimally invasive and relatively inexpensive, even though it would likely not be warranted in most people who present with acute bacterial sinusitis.

In some cases, a physician might elect to conduct an empirical trial of treatment for a suspected condition instead of opting for diagnostic testing. However, in the case of CVID, the testing for the condition is relatively inexpensive, whereas treatment is not. Thus, in this particular case, it is probably better to have more decision support for treatment (in terms of a positive serum test) than to elect to conduct an empirical trial without further testing.

Testing for CVID involves measuring the levels of immunoglobulin G (IgG; and sometimes IgM and IgA) in the serum. If the levels are low, then the patient is treated with replacement IgG, generally either monthly intravenously or weekly subcutaneously, at a cost, in most cases (depending on dose), of more than $100,000 per year. Because of the difficulty and expense in treating CVID, the physician in this example will want to be as confident as possible in the diagnosis. Although all medical diagnoses are at some level uncertain, physicians must be confident that they are at least "approaching a solution" before initiating treatment (Barrows and Pickell 1991), particularly if, as in this case, the treatment involves significant expense.

Because of the inherent uncertainty of the diagnostic process, there is always the potential for missed or mistaken diagnosis in clinical practice, and all physicians need to be aware of this. Because of this potential for diagnostic mistakes, some have argued that we might have more confidence in our diagnoses if computer-based diagnostic algorithms were used more regularly. There are currently many diagnostic programs either available or in development, and dozens of studies have compared computer-aided diagnosis with expert diagnosis. However, whether such programs could eventually replace human diagnosticians is still under debate in the medical and computer science literature. Although some of these studies show that computer-aided diagnoses outperform expert diagnoses in certain settings (Grove 2000), they have not yet gained widespread use in the clinical setting.

Let us suppose that the physician in our example, given the patient history and presentation, decides to test for total IgG and finds that the IgG level is 530 mg/dL (the normal value is 700 to 1,600 mg/dL). What does this mean for the patient's diagnosis? In order to answer this question, the test information needs to be used to estimate the post-test probability of CVID. In other words, in our particular example, the physician must ask, "What is the probability of CVID given a total IgG level of less than 700 and a history of frequent bacterial sinusitis?" The answer to this question in turn depends on an evaluation of both pre- and post-test probability of the disease. This can be done informally, which is what is usually the case in clinical practice, or formally, using Bayes' theorem. Bayes' theorem is a mathematical formula that is used to calculate post-test probabilities given pretest probability and new evidence (e.g., a test result). For instance, Bayes' theorem can be used to determine the probability that a person who tests positive for CVID actually has the disease. Specifically, in our example, we are interested in the probability of a person having CVID (X), if he has a positive test result $(+)$.

According to Bayes' theorem, this probability is:

$$\Pr(X \mid +) = [\Pr(X) \times \Pr(+ \mid X)] / \Pr(+)$$

Let us assume that a positive test result for CVID is indicated by an IgG level of 700 or less and that the occurrence of the disease in the general population is .004 percent. Furthermore, for the sake of illustration, let us also assume the following values, which represent the features of the test:

Pr (positive test result | subject has CVID) = 96%
Pr (negative test result | subject has CVID) = 4%
Pr (negative test result | subject does not have CVID) = 91%
Pr (positive test result | subject does not have CVID) = 9%

First, we need to find $\Pr(+)$. This is given by

$$\Pr(+) = [\Pr(+ \mid X) \times \Pr(X)] + [\Pr(+ \mid \sim X) \times \Pr(\sim X)]$$

where X is the occurrence of the disease in the general population, + is a positive test result, and $\sim X$ is the probability that someone in the general population does not have CVID. Substituting in our previous numbers, we get

$$\Pr(+) = [.96 \times .00004] + [.09 \times .99996] = .0900348$$

Now we can substitute the calculated value of Pr(+) into our formulation of Bayes' theorem:

$$Pr(X \mid +) = (.00004 \times .96) / .0900348 = .0004265$$

This result shows us that even with a positive test result for CVID, it is very unlikely that a person randomly chosen from the general population has the disease. However, the probability that the patient in our example (given a positive test result) has CVID is not the same as the probability (calculated previously) of a person in the general population (given a positive test result) having it. The diagnosis of CVID in this particular patient depends largely on his history of frequent, recurrent bacterial infections, which is used to determine the pretest probability of the disease. In other words, this particular information from the patient's medical history makes it far more likely that he, compared to a randomly chosen individual from the general population, has CVID.

This dependence of diagnosis on other pieces of evidence aside from test results highlights the clinical and diagnostic importance of carefully conducting the patient interview and patient examination. This is because the pretest probability is not created in a vacuum— it is patient-specific (and physician-specific). In other words, a diagnosis cannot ever be made on the basis of test results alone. No test, however accurate, is ever 100 percent accurate. More important, a probabilistic determination of the likelihood of disease in a given patient is not just a matter of crunching numbers. Instead, the probability that a patient has the disease in question in any given case will always depend, at least in part, on nonstatistical evidence such as the medical history and/or patient examination. Here again, as in all areas of medical practice, ethics is intertwined with evidence: In order to gather a thorough patient history, as previously discussed, a physician must learn to listen to the patient, not just in order to "be nice" but because accurate diagnosis depends on it.

3.6. TREATMENT PLANNING

Once a diagnosis is made, the physician can then turn their attention to formulating, together with the patient, a plan for treating the diagnosed condition. This plan must consider the financial cost and risks/side effects, on the one hand, and the potential benefits of the proposed treatment, on the other hand. In our example, the treatment is very high in cost but carries little risk and a high potential for patient benefit. With regard to treatment decisions, it is generally understood that the patient has the final decision-making authority and can choose whether or not to accept or reject a proposed treatment plan. However, decisional *priority* might lie with the physician, the patient, or both (Whitney 2003). This means that in some cases, a patient might wish to defer a treatment (or a diagnostic) decision to their physician. However, in many cases, patients want to participate with their physicians in the decision-making process. The concept of shared decision-making is much discussed in current medical literature. Although it is agreed that sharing the burden of decision-making is best for both patients and physicians, exactly how this should be done in practice is much debated.

For instance, one might wonder whether or not patients should be given all the relevant information about various testing and treatment options or whether instead physicians should narrow down these choices according to their own expertise and preferences before presenting them to their patients. On the one hand, it is argued that patient autonomy depends on completeness of information. On the other hand, it has been noted that patient satisfaction "has been shown to be higher when people choose from a smaller set of options" (Botti and Iyengar 2004, p. 324), perhaps because too many options can seem overwhelming to patients when they feel that they do not have enough education or information to make an intelligent choice from among the options. Furthermore, some have argued that giving patients too much information about the risks or side effects of a treatment option could harm patients by causing them to forgo treatment that would be beneficial to their health goals. Thus, both giving and withholding medical information can have consequences, and when weighing this, the physician needs to consider the patient's goals and desires. Although patient satisfaction is not the sole goal of clinical medicine, it is nevertheless clearly something that needs to be taken into account during the process of medical decision-making and thus cannot be ignored.

Furthermore, although accurate information must be given to a patient before the patient can make an informed decision regarding a diagnostic or a treatment option, "precise information (e.g., about risk) is frequently ineffective in changing decisions and behaviors" because patients and professionals rely on the personally relevant *meaning* of the information rather than on the information itself (Reyna 2008, p. 855). In other words, although it is important that patients are told what their options are, physicians must also allow them the opportunity to interpret these options according to their own values and preferences because this is the only way to facilitate truly informed consent. Once this interpretation has taken place and been discussed, the physician and the patient can then decide together upon a mutually agreeable course of action.

In our example, if the patient is diagnosed with CVID, then the patient and the physician will have to decide together how best to treat the condition. In some cases, if the infections are mild enough (i.e., if they do not require, for instance, intravenous antibiotics or extended hospital visits), the physician might suggest trying pro-phylactic antibiotic therapy before moving to IgG replacement. The benefit of continuous antibiotic treatment is that it is less expen-sive than either intravenous or subcutaneous IgG; however, there are disadvantages to this option as well. First, although antibiotics might work to prevent bacterial infections such as the sinusitis this patient had been experiencing, they do not prevent viral or para-sitic infections—infections that CVID patients are also predis-posed to getting. Second, long-term antibiotic therapy can lead to reduced and/or changed intestinal flora, with resulting decreased immunity to certain infections—clearly not a benefit to someone who is already immune deficient. Third, long-term treatment with antibiotics can result in antibiotic-resistant organisms, which might be passed to others in the community.

On the other hand, IgG therapy, although not entailing the disadvantages of continuous antibiotic therapy, has its own risks. The most significant risks of IgG therapy are blood clots and other complications due to hyperviscosity (Katz et al. 2007). Furthermore, IgG treatment is both expensive and inconvenient. Intravenous IgG must be given either in an infusion center or by a home health care practitioner and takes four to six hours per infu-sion, one day per month. For the patient, this means a potential loss of one full workday per month if an infusion center or home health care practitioner with weekend hours is not available. In that case, subcutaneous IgG therapy might be a better option. Although sub-cutaneous IgG is generally more expensive than intravenous IgG, it can be administered by the patient at home (without assistance) on a weekly basis. Infusion time for this method of delivery ranges from one to three hours per infusion. Some patients, however, are not willing or able to self-infuse, so this option cannot be utilized in all cases.

3.7. CONCLUSION

As demonstrated by the analysis of the example presented in this chapter, even in patient cases that might initially appear to be relatively uncomplicated, the process of DDM can be very complex, and in all instances, it involves considerations of epistemology (e.g., how to understand diagnostic information), ethics (e.g., consideration of patient values and preferences or of how much information to give a patient in order to facilitate informed consent), probability (e.g., when interpreting diagnostic test results), and economics. Furthermore, the process of DDM is patient-specific both in terms of qualitative evidence toward a diagnosis (e.g., information from the medical history) and in terms of quantitative evidence (e.g., pre- and post-test probabilities). Thus, learning to make diagnostic decisions requires at least a basic understanding of concepts in each of these fields as well as careful consideration on the part of both the physician and the patient as to how these considerations bear on the individual case at hand. In addition, it requires a commitment on the part of each to shared decision-making in the clinical context.

Chapter 4

Handling Uncertainty

4.1. BACKGROUND

Based on the discussion of diagnostic decision-making in Chapter 3, it is no secret that medical practice—from testing methods to diagnostic reasoning, treatment protocols, and prognostic evaluations—is often both complex and uncertain. What this means in practice is that it is not always possible to determine the precise cause of a patient's signs and symptoms, to know for certain how to treat those signs and symptoms, or to accurately predict how they will (or will not) progress. This general and pervasive uncertainty in medicine is well recognized in both medical and philosophical literature (Fox 1957; Atkinson 1984; Upshur 2000; Djulbegovic, Hozo, and Greenland 2011; Simpkin and Schwartzstein 2016). Fox (1957), in particular, describes medical uncertainty as taking three distinct forms:

> The first results from incomplete or imperfect mastery of available knowledge. No one can have at his command all skills and all knowledge of the lore of medicine. The second depends upon limitations in current medical knowledge. There are innumerable questions to which no physician, however well trained, can

as yet provide answers. A third source of uncertainty derives from the first two. This consists of difficulty in distinguishing between personal ignorance or ineptitude and the limitations of present medical knowledge. (pp. 208–209)

This means that no medical practitioner can ever be completely immune to encountering uncertainty: Even if the practitioner masters all of the available medical knowledge, there will always be limitations upon that knowledge. But this does not need to be cause for despair. Rather, instead of fearing diagnostic uncertainty or, worse, pretending that it does not exist, physicians can be trained to recognize it, and to effectively manage it, in the clinical setting.

The discussion of diagnostic uncertainty in this chapter proceeds via the examination of several case studies, all of which were purposefully chosen because I consider them to be ordinary, or routine, and not in any way unusual. I focus on these routine cases because they are of the sort that are regularly encountered by physicians in their everyday work and thus highlight the fact that diagnostic uncertainty is not reserved for strange, unusual, or otherwise fantastic cases, as is sometimes wrongly assumed. In what follows, I attempt both to explain why there is often diagnostic uncertainty even in routine cases and to make some suggestions as to how this uncertainty can be helpfully mitigated, or at least managed, in the clinical setting. The first example case shows how a mishandling of diagnostic uncertainty has the potential to lead to premature closure of a medical case and thus to potentially cause both medical and ethical harm. The second case serves to highlight the dangers of dismissing diagnostic uncertainty, and the third case shows what can happen when diagnostic uncertainty is blamed on the patient. In cases such as these three, both diagnostic accuracy and physician–patient interaction could be improved via the recognition of and the communication (to the patient) of medical uncertainty during the process of differential diagnosis.

4.2. CASE 1: ABDOMINAL PAIN

A 67-year-old man was sent by ambulance from his assisted living home to the emergency department (ED) of a large research hospital with the chief complaint of ongoing diarrhea and abdominal pain. Abdominal pain is notoriously nonspecific and can indicate any number of conditions of varying degrees of severity; thus, it requires a careful workup when it presents in the emergency setting. This particular case was especially complicated because the man had a previous history of prostate cancer. Because of this, he had developed incontinence, which required self-catheterization several times per day. Furthermore, the self-catheterization had in turn led to frequent urinary tract infections (UTIs). More complicated still, this man had also recently developed a *Clostridium difficile* infection secondary to antibiotic treatment for a UTI, yet it was unclear from the patient's history whether or not the treatment for the *C. difficile* infection was successful, as he reported that he continued to have chronic diarrhea and stomach pain (which could have been indicative of a persistent infection) even after finishing the prescribed course of antibiotic treatment. Finally, to add even more complication to the case, it was not clear when the diarrhea had initially started, as the patient's hospital record indicated that it had been ongoing for several years. Because of this complex history, the patient's symptoms could not be definitely attributed to *C. difficile* and yet that diagnosis could not be absolutely ruled out either.

After the patient's history was taken, the attending physician ordered a urinalysis and a computed tomography (CT) of the abdomen to be performed. The urinalysis showed seven white blood cells (which are not normally present in healthy urine), indicating that a UTI was a possibility, and the CT scan showed several metastatic masses, indicating that cancer could also be a potential cause of the patient's symptoms. Hospital records showed that the same masses were visible on a CT scan that had been taken on a previous hospital admission three months earlier, indicating that there had not been significant recent growth of the masses. Given these historical- and test-based findings, the man was given a differential diagnosis of UTI versus infectious diarrhea versus cancer versus gastritis. The man did not have fever or diarrhea while he was in the ED, so the diagnosis of infectious diarrhea (caused by C. difficile or a virus or some other organism) was difficult to rule in or out because a stool analysis could not be performed and no clear, definitive signs of infection were present.

4.3. CASE ANALYSIS

This case is representative of many others like it in the following respect: None of the presenting evidence (including the history and the laboratory and other findings) was such that it allowed for definitively ruling out any of the diagnoses in the initial differential list. In other words, the diagnosis in this case was very clearly epistemically uncertain: It could not be determined, at least initially, whether the man's symptoms were due to infectious diarrhea, UTI, cancer, or something else. This case also makes a good study because the diagnostic uncertainty it displays is relatively easy to recognize. Nevertheless, the uncertainty still became problematic in this case. Hospital records indicated that the patient had reported the same symptoms of diarrhea and abdominal pain at both his first and second admissions to the ED, three months apart. Furthermore, an abdominal CT and a stool culture were performed during his first admission, and at that time the stool culture was positive for C. difficile. The patient was informed of this result and was given a prescription for oral antibiotic treatment for this infectious condition. The hospital record indicated that the official diagnosis for the patient's complaints at that time was "infectious diarrhea due to C. difficile."

However, neither the man nor his gastroenterologist was informed of the results of the CT scan, and it is not clear whether this was an oversight that was directly or indirectly related to the diagnostic uncertainty of the case. In any case, on the patient's subsequent visit to the ED three months later, the new attending physician immediately recognized the uncertainty inherent in the previous diagnosis and instead of diagnosing the man with recurrent or undertreated C. difficile, he reopened the diagnostic differential and re-examined all of the available evidence. It was because of this that he found the CT scan results from the previous admission. After finding them, the attending physician spent a long time deliberating over what to do because he had to decide whether to admit the patient to the hospital or to send him back to the assisted living home. After deliberation, the physician decided not to treat the patient for a suspected UTI, given the history of C. difficile that had occurred subsequent to previous antibiotic treatment for that condition. Instead, the physician sent the urine out for culture. He decided that given that the immediate risk to the patient from any of the conditions in the differential was low, he could safely suspend judgment on the patient's case while conducting further investigation. So he sent the man home with instructions to follow up with his gastroenterologist the next week. Finally, the physician also indicated on the patient's discharge instructions that he should be treated for a UTI if bacteria were cultured from the urine sample.

Suspending judgment, as this physician did, on a diagnostically uncertain case is often the best course of action for several reasons. First, making diagnoses on the basis of insufficient evidence, rather than suspending judgment, is likely to lead to missed or misdiagnosis (Kennedy 2013), whereas suspending judgment on a case can allow, as it did in this one, for continued investigation into the cause of the illness in question. In other words, suspending judgment does not have to result in paralysis or inaction. Instead, there is the possibility for action even before a definitive diagnosis is made, and one form that this can take, aside from promoting further investigation, is that of accepting a "working diagnosis." Accepting a working diagnosis is an "evaluative response" that allows the physician to act without requiring belief in any of the initial diagnostic hypotheses (Elliott and Willmes 2013). This means, for example, that when a physician accepts a diagnosis as a basis for action, the physician does not need to believe that the diagnosis is correct, accurate, or permanent but can instead simply use the diagnosis on a trial basis. One way that this is often implemented in practice is with the use of an "empirical trial," which involves giving a treatment for one of the conditions in the differential to determine if the patient responds. If the patient responds to the treatment, this is evidence that the patient has the condition in question. Thus, "observing a patient's response (or lack of response) to empiric therapy can provide valuable diagnostic information" (Brett and Powell 2011, p. 18). This means that, at least in some cases, a physician can arrive at a definitive diagnosis by accepting a tentative one.

In fact, many diagnoses are, at least initially, tentative. There are very few cases in which it is appropriate to call a diagnosis "certain." This is because a diagnosis is a hypothesis, the evidence for which can vary greatly in degree. Thus, the cognitive attitude that a physician should take toward many (and possibly even most) diagnoses is one of acceptance for the purposes of further action, rather than of belief that the diagnosis is correct, definitive, or true.

Second, suspending judgment on a case both requires and allows for an honest communication of the diagnostic uncertainty to the patient and thereby promotes a respectful consideration of the patient as an active participant on the health care team.

There are several reasons why this kind of epistemic honesty is beneficial in clinical practice. First, it encourages physicians to take the patient's symptoms seriously and to refrain from being dismissive of the patient's self-report in difficult-to-diagnose cases. Second, it also encourages physicians to keep the diagnostic differential open to revision and to thereby avoid the dangers of the overconfidence bias. Berner and Graber (2008), who have written on this bias, argue that "physicians in general underappreciate that their diagnoses are wrong" (p. S2). One of the dangers inherent with an overconfidence bias is that it can lead to a breakdown in clinical reasoning, and thus an overconfident physician might have problems gathering data, such as by failing to elicit complete and accurate information from the patient; failing to recognize the significance of data, such as misinterpreting test results; or, most commonly, failing to synthesize or "put it all together" (p. S8).

Another danger with an overconfidence bias is that it tends to lead to definitive, and potentially dangerous, action in the face of uncertainty. In fact, it has been found that the greater the epistemic uncertainty of the diagnostic situation, the more likely physicians are to exercise overconfidence in the clinic (Croskerry and Norman

2008). Thus, what comes naturally to many physicians when they are faced with uncertainty is exactly the opposite of what is called for by best diagnostic practice. Instead of definitive action that closes off further investigation, best diagnostic practice, in many cases, calls for the physician to either adopt a working diagnosis or leave the investigation open while further evidence is being gathered.

Interestingly, however, although most physicians are willing to admit that medicine is, in general, an uncertain practice, they rarely acknowledge the uncertainty inherent in *their own* day-to-day practice: "Although physicians are rationally aware when uncertainty exists, the culture of medicine evinces a deep-rooted unwillingness to acknowledge and embrace it" (Simpkin and Schwartzstein 2016, p. 1713). This is very likely due in large part to the enormous societal pressure put on physicians (by their patients and others) to always have the "right answers," right away. However, explicit training in the recognition, management, and pervasiveness of diagnostic uncertainty during medical school, residency, and fellowship can help remedy these sorts of reactions to this undue pressure.

Early in my teaching career, I was surprised to learn that most U.S. medical schools and residency programs do not offer (much less require) a formal course in diagnostic reasoning (Rencic et al. 2017). Given the importance of diagnostic reasoning in clinical practice, clearly it would be beneficial to change this situation (and indeed that is one motivation for writing this book). In addition, such a potential change seems to be supported by the vast majority of practicing physicians as well as medical school professors, who report that they think that diagnostic reasoning should be taught, in a more formal way than it currently is taught, to medical students and trainees. The cited reason for why this is not generally done is "lack of faculty expertise" (Rencic et al. 2017). I suspect, however, that many medical school faculty as well as residency directors are in fact very well qualified to teach diagnostic reasoning but that because it has not been traditionally part of the curriculum in these programs, it has continued to be neglected.

Returning to our case study, the attending physician during the patient's second ED visit did in fact recognize the uncertainty in the situation that the first treatment team had missed. He handled it initially by deciding to suspend judgment until more information could be gathered. But then he faced the difficult question of how to communicate his findings and recommendations to his patient. What made the situation especially difficult is that it was clear from the initial conversation between the two, which I witnessed, that the patient was hoping for a solution to, or at least a definitive explanation for, his symptoms. In other words, he wanted, as nearly all patients do, an answer from the doctor that would explain his symptoms. In fact, the patient had explicitly expressed frustration at his ongoing undiagnosed symptoms and multiple ED visits and clearly wanted to know the cause of his continuing suffering. The most difficult part of the attending physician's management of this case was that he could not provide what the patient wanted: He did not have a definitive answer to give the man concerning the cause of his long-standing symptoms. The physician could have chosen to act as if he did have a definitive answer, but instead, he consciously decided (after much deliberation!) to be honest in his conversation with the patient and to tell him that he simply did not know what was causing the continuing abdominal pain and diarrhea. He did this by approaching the patient and simply stating, "I don't know what is causing your pain, but I am working on finding out."

The patient was clearly surprised to hear the physician admit his uncertainty, yet he expressed his appreciation for the physician's honesty. The physician later told me, privately, that in more than twenty years of medical practice, he had never admitted to any patient, ever, that he "did not know." That day marked the very first time that he had ever said those words aloud to any patient. This, in itself, is very telling of the enormous societal pressure placed upon physicians to have all the answers and to get everything right all the time, which is both unrealistic and potentially dangerous: "Physicians' difficulty in accepting uncertainty has also been associated with detrimental effects on patients, including excessive ordering of tests that carry risks of false positive results or iatrogenic injury and withholding of information from patients" (Simpkin and Schwartzstein 2016, p. 1713). Given these risks, together with the fact that diagnostic uncertainty is pervasive, more should be done to train physicians to recognize, manage, and communicate diagnostic uncertainty effectively to their patients when it is present.

In this particular case, the communication of diagnostic uncertainty to the patient went over well. One could certainly imagine, however, a case in which a patient might not appreciate honesty concerning the uncertainty of their diagnosis. Patients are individuals; as such, it should be acknowledged that uncertainty can be very uncomfortable for some and that therefore it should be communicated thoughtfully and, at times, delicately. But it should always be communicated and never hidden. There are two reasons for this. The first is an ethical one: Being honest with a patient is always better than the alternative. The second is a medical/scientific one: When uncertainty is ignored, medical outcomes are the worse for it. Thus, uncertainty in a diagnostic case should always be communicated to the patient. However, when doing so, a physician should be aware of how the patient is receiving the news. Some patients, for example, will want very detailed information about their case, whereas others will not. The key to effective communication of uncertainty in diagnosis is to carefully consider the needs of the individual patient and to always couple the news of the uncertainty with an assurance that the physician will continue to investigate the case until a more definitive diagnosis can be made. Then, of course, the physician must follow through on this assurance.

Also note that in this case, the patient's prior visit to the ED had proceeded quite differently. Although the presenting evidence at that time had also rendered the case diagnostically uncertain (he was found to have both a C. *difficile* infection and metastatic masses in the abdomen), the team that initially managed the patient's case settled on a definitive diagnosis of infectious diarrhea as the cause of the patient's symptoms, without communicating the uncertainty of the situation to the patient or his gastroenterologist. Again, the reasons for this are not clear. But whatever the reason for the mishandling of this case, it put both the patient (for health reasons) and the hospital (for legal reasons) at risk of significant harm. Because the diagnosis of C. *difficile* was definitively recorded in the patient's chart, no further investigation into the cause of his abdominal pain and diarrhea was conducted by the physicians that the patient saw in the interim between his two hospital visits. In other words, the case was prematurely closed as a consequence of the lack of recognition and acknowledgment of the uncertainty in the initial diagnosis. Ultimately, this cost the patient many months of suffering as well as multiple ED and clinic visits. It might have even shortened his life because what was missed in this case was cancer.

Many lessons can be learned from an examination of this case. The first is that settling too quickly on a single diagnosis is not in the best medical interest of the patient even when the patient (and/ or the physician) is clearly hoping for a definitive answer to or solution for the presenting symptoms. Instead, a willingness to suspend judgment in the face of an uncertain diagnostic situation, and thus to keep open the scientific investigation into the cause of a patient's complaints, is preferable to too quickly settling on a single diagnosis in the face of underdetermining evidence. There are other reasons as well. During the man's first ED admission, the attending physician might have reasoned that given the man's age, the metastatic masses found on the abdominal CT were unlikely to be of immediate harm and that informing the man of their presence would not be of any therapeutic benefit. Thus, the uncertainty in this case might have been ignored because the other conditions in the diagnostic differential were not considered to be of appreciable risk to the patient. There are, of course, good, practical, reasons for treating high-risk and/or immediate dangers first. Certainly, treating the man's *C. difficile* infection, which was an immediate risk, was appropriate. But one error, at least, in this case was that the uncertainty in the diagnosis was not acknowledged, nor was it communicated, and thus the cancer that was found on the man's CT scan was never investigated. Instead, only the *C. difficile* diagnosis was communicated to the man and recorded in the hospital record.

4.4. CASE 2: CHEST PAIN AND SHORTNESS OF BREATH

A 29-year-old man was admitted to the ED of another major hospital [pre-coronavirus disease 2019 (COVID-19)] with the chief complaint of chest pain and shortness of breath. He denied any history of allergies or asthma. Upon examination, he was found to have a productive cough, which produced green sputum, and significant difficulty with breathing. The family members who had driven him to the hospital made a specific request that the man be given antibiotic therapy for his condition. However, because chest imaging was negative for pneumonia, the attending physician denied this request, concluding that the man had a viral upper respiratory infection. He then treated the patient with albuterol. Fifteen minutes after the albuterol treatment, the patient reported easier breathing but continued to look quite ill. The physician explained to the man that he had a bad cold, that he definitely did not need antibiotics, and that his condition would improve on its own without treatment.

4.5. CASE ANALYSIS

This sort of case is very commonly seen in both the emergency and primary care settings, and yet it is still often handled inappropriately, as it was in this instance. In this particular case, the patient displayed symptoms (difficulty breathing and productive cough with green sputum) that are consistent with both viral and bacterial respiratory tract infection, and thus the diagnosis of a viral infection in this case, and in many like it, was inherently uncertain because the evidence was underdetermining. There is no way to simply look at a patient and determine by physical examination alone whether or not the patient has a viral or bacterial respiratory tract infection. It is possible, however, to home in on the probability of viral versus bacterial infection in any given case by taking a careful patient history. As discussed in Chapter 3, it is well known that in the general population viral upper respiratory infections are more common than bacterial ones. However, this statistic does not apply to all individual cases. Instead, in patients with a history of recurrent bacterial respiratory infection, that condition is more common than the former.

Nevertheless, in this case, the patient was not informed of this diagnostic uncertainty, nor was he questioned about a history of previous bacterial respiratory infections. Instead, he was told that his infection was definitely caused by a virus. That made his diagnosis both epistemically and ethically problematic. The diagnosis was epistemically problematic because the evidence that was gathered was insufficient to support it. Furthermore, it was ethically problematic because it led the physician to be dismissive of the patient's illness, by not communicating the epistemic situation to him. Given the presenting evidence in this case, it was not possible to make a definitive determination between the two possible diagnoses (bacterial vs. viral respiratory infection). However, the attending physician did not even entertain the hypothesis that the patient's infection was bacterial, even though the evidence was consistent with this. If he had entertained this possibility, or perhaps had used it as a working diagnosis, the physician might have cultured the patient's sputum or considered an empirical trial of antibiotic therapy, thereby keeping the investigation into the cause of the patient's symptoms open. Even if the diagnosis of viral infection turned out to be correct, making this diagnosis, without either considering or informing the patient of the possibility that the illness was bacterial instead of viral, was harmful to the patient for two reasons. First, it was harmful because it prematurely closed the investigation into the cause of the patient's illness, possibly resulting in misdiagnosis. Second, it was harmful because it was dismissive of the patient's concerns. Telling the patient that he had a cold and did not need antibiotics might have been true. But it might have been false. In this case, the risk of long-term physical harm to the patient because of misdiagnosis was low because he was young and in relatively good health. If he did have a bacterial infection, and not a viral one, this infection could likely be safely treated at a later time if symptoms persisted. Although delaying the proper treatment of the infection would have caused some extra suffering (and perhaps missed days of work) for the patient, it is unlikely that it would have posed a serious or long-term risk to his health. But this is not always the case: In some situations, misdiagnosis can be serious or even fatal. Ignoring diagnostic uncertainty in routine cases should thus be avoided because it can lead to a tendency to also ignore uncertainty in more serious cases. Therefore, even in cases in which the risk to the patient is perceived by the physician to be low, diagnostic uncertainty should not be ignored.

A complicating factor in this particular case is the issue of antibiotic resistance. The problem of antibiotic resistance is real and growing. According to the Centers for Disease Control and Prevention (2020), approximately 700,000 people die from antibiotic-resistant infections each year. Furthermore, every year, new multidrug-resistant organisms emerge. Because of this, health care professionals are advised not to prescribe antibiotics to patients unless they are absolutely needed. But this, of course, does not mean that physicians should automatically assume that all low-risk cases are not bacterial, or that they do not require antibiotic treatment. It is a diagnostic pitfall to make the assumption that because there is an ethical concern related to a specific treatment for a particular condition, that condition ought not to be diagnosed or should be diagnosed less frequently. The frequency of occurrence of disease, or the likelihood that any given patient might have it, is of course independent of any considerations of its treatment. Thus, the diagnosis of a condition should occur independently from treatment considerations. In other words, a physician should never withhold a diagnosis from a patient based on concerns regarding how the diagnosed condition might be treated, because this can lead, in some cases, to serious, detrimental consequences.

4.6. CASE 3: ADDISON'S DISEASE

As a third example, consider the following case report:

A 41-year-old man who worked in construction presented to our psychiatric clinic complaining of depressed mood that had started two months previously. He related his condition to the recent and violent loss of his spouse, who was killed in a car accident. The patient's symptoms included loss of concentration, lack of sleep, and loss of appetite leading to a six-pound weight loss over the previous two months. He denied any suicidal thoughts but admitted that he sometimes heard his spouse's voice in the house. After discussing the condition as a case of depression with the patient, we started the patient on psychotherapy sessions (twice monthly) and 20 mg of fluoxetine daily. The patient came to the clinic for follow-up two weeks later. He complained that the therapy had done nothing to improve his mood and that he thought, in fact, his condition was worsening. He stated that two days previously, he thought he saw his deceased spouse in the kitchen. He also reported having thoughts about death and the futility of life without his partner, although he insisted he was not suicidal and that he had no plans for committing suicide. We advised the patient to continue taking the fluoxetine, and we increased his psychotherapy sessions to weekly. After this follow-up visit, the patient, however, only attended one psychotherapy session and was lost to follow-up for several months. Four months later, the patient presented to our emergency room (ER) with delirium, mild fever, and visual and auditory hallucinations. According to the ER team, the provisional diagnosis was substance abuse, but the toxicology screen came back negative, denying this diagnosis. The treatment team noted a weak, thready pulse, severe hypotension

(70 systolic), and severe hyponatremia and hyperkalemia. A diagnosis of an Addisonian crisis was made. The patient was admitted to the intensive care unit, and proper intervention for the Addisonian crisis was administered. Later, it came to our attention that the patient had visited several physicians and hospitals in the area during the past four months, but a diagnosis of Addison's disease was not made by anyone (Abdel-Motleb 2012).

Addison's disease, or primary adrenal insufficiency, is an endocrine disorder that is characterized by the decreased output of steroids (including cortisol, aldosterone, and dehydroepiandosterone) from the adrenal cortex. It occurs in all age groups and affects both sexes. It can be caused by hemorrhage, injury, infection, or autoimmune destruction of the adrenal tissue. Symptoms of this disease include severe fatigue, muscle weakness, loss of appetite, weight loss, nausea, irritability, depression, low blood pressure, hypoglycemia, sleep disturbance, hyperpigmentation, and increased susceptibility to infection. If left untreated, it can result in death due to the inability to mount a sufficient cortisol response to daily stressors. Addison's disease can be diagnosed either by the detection of a low morning cortisol level in the blood or by an impaired response to an adrenocorticotropic hormone (ACTH) stimulation test (Dorin, Qualls, and Crapo 2003). In a healthy subject, this exogenous stimulation with a synthetic form of the pituitary hormone ACTH results in a significant cortisol increase over baseline. However, in a patient with Addison's disease, the stimulation response is either low or nonexistent. Addison's disease, once it is detected, can be treated by replacing the hormones that the adrenal glands cannot make. These treatments are both readily available and relatively inexpensive.

Addison's disease is not common and therefore is only rarely encountered in the clinical setting. It is estimated that Addison's disease occurs with a frequency of only approximately 39 to 140 per 1 million (Lovas and Husebye 2002). Because of its infrequency, the diagnosis of the disease is often either delayed or missed. Missed diagnosis of Addison's disease usually occurs because the presenting symptoms are nonspecific and are commonly associated with depression or anxiety. In fact, more than 68 percent of Addison's disease patients are initially given an incorrect diagnosis, usually of depression or hypochondria (Hiroi et al. 2010). Although several journal articles have warned that "physicians must be aware that Addison's disease may present solely with psychiatric symptoms and maintain a high index of suspicion for this potentially fatal condition" (Hiroi et al. 2010, p. 56) and have further suggested that "blood work for ACTH and cortisol in the field of psychiatry" should be employed (Iwata et al. 2004, p. 1112), the rate of missed diagnosis of this disease remains high.

4.7. CASE ANALYSIS

In this case, the patient initially presented in the clinic with symptoms consistent with depression (or at least with normal grief due to bereavement) subsequent to the traumatic loss of his spouse. Given this history and presentation, the initial diagnosis of depression seems appropriate. However, the patient returned to the clinic two weeks later, complaining that his symptoms had worsened. This should have been the first clue to the examining physicians that something was amiss and that further investigation into the patient's case was warranted. Although it is true that more than two weeks are required to observe the full therapeutic effects of treatment with a selective serotonin reuptake inhibitor such as fluoxetine, symptoms usually do not worsen once treatment has begun. Thus, the patient's report that he was worsening should have prompted further investigation on the part of the physicians—perhaps with a more detailed medical history or with another physical examination. So why didn't the physicians do this? One possible reason is that they were simply thinking pragmatically. According to currently accepted evidence-based medicine guidelines, not all clinical problems are considered worthy of the time and effort necessary for their solution (Sackett et al. 2000, p. 198). In practical terms, this means that, among other things, physicians must decide whether or not it is time- and cost-effective to evaluate their patients with laboratory or other testing procedures or with repeated clinical examinations. In making this decision, the physician must take into consideration the likelihood that the patient has a serious, treatable disease. Addison's disease is both serious and treatable, but it is uncommon, and this is probably why it was not initially suspected in this patient's case. After all, a patient who has just lost a spouse seems far more likely to have clinical depression than to have Addison's disease. Thus, the problem in this case was not primarily with the initial diagnosis. Rather, the problem was that the patient's symptom severity was dismissed on his repeated visits to several physicians and hospitals. At some point, one of the examining physicians should have questioned the initial diagnosis. However, as far as can be seen from the details of this case report, no one did. Thus, the diagnostic pitfall in this case was that the patient's own reports of worsening were not given sufficient weight as being relevant—until it was nearly too late. This is of course the sort of diagnostic situation that physicians should try to avoid.

Instead, physicians should practice a compassionate suspension of judgment in the clinical setting when the patient's illness cannot be immediately diagnosed. There are three reasons in support of this. Suspending judgment in this way (1) encourages ongoing investigation, (2) promotes epistemic humility, and (3) shows respect for the patient.

Suppose that, in this case, instead of prematurely closing the scientific investigation, the physicians had decided to suspend judgment about the cause of the patient's continued, worsening symptoms. According to Martinez (2012), this would have encouraged further investigation. He argues that "uncertainty . . . propels activity—doctors have a propensity to resolve uncertainty and ambiguity by action rather than inaction" (p. 17). The action propelled by uncertainty that would have resulted if the physicians had suspended judgment in this case would thus have had a methodological benefit: The physicians who examined the patient on his repeated visits would have been more likely to discover the actual cause of the patient's symptoms. It might be objected here that pragmatic considerations, such as the time and monetary costs involved in further investigation in this case, would take precedence over any methodological benefit gained. In other words, it might be objected that if a suspension of judgment encourages further investigation, then it should *not* be preferred—because it would be too costly in terms of both time and money. Although it is true that research and testing can be both time-consuming and expensive, and that this is a consideration that every physician must take into account when deciding how to act in the clinical setting, it should not be assumed that dismissing a patient's concerns, rather than continuing investigation, is always less costly. For example, in this case, significant amounts of time and money (on repeated hospital visits and unnecessary medication) were wasted. For this and other reasons, physicians should not be too quick to allow pragmatic considerations to prevent them from reopening investigation into a case when new evidence arises.

In addition, Martinez (2012) warns that physicians should take care not to allow intellectual laziness to "pass for pragmatism." In cases in which a physician is not able to make an immediate diagnosis, the physician has "to want to know what's going on" (Guram, 2011, p. 14) in order to proceed effectively and avoid diagnostic mistakes. In other words, in order to be a good physician, one must be intellectually curious—and this is promoted in the clinical setting not by dismissing the patient's concerns but, rather, by the suspension of judgment when an immediate diagnosis cannot be made.

We have seen that suspending judgment in the clinical setting, in cases in which an immediate diagnosis cannot be made, often leads to further investigation, which in turn increases the chances of correct diagnosis. Furthermore, it also encourages epistemic humility. Because every physician is continually faced with uncertainty, Schwab (2012) argues that physicians must be prepared to decide how they will handle it when it arises. This of course first requires *recognizing* it, which in turn requires repeated and regular self-reflection. If uncertainty is not handled appropriately by the physician, it can cause significant harm to the patient by causing a diagnosis to be delayed inappropriately or missed entirely. In this particular case, the physicians were uncertain as to whether there was physical disease present in the patient, and because of this they dismissed the patient's reports of worsening illness instead of suspending judgment while continuing investigation into the cause of the patient's complaints. Thus, in so doing, the physicians displayed a lack of epistemic humility, which was ultimately harmful for the patient in question. Epistemic humility (Schwab 2012) is a characteristic of claims that accurately portray the quality of evidence for believing the claims to be accurate. In other words, epistemically humble claims neither overreach nor underreach the evidence that supports them. In this particular case, the epistemic error was ignoring further evidence in the patient's history once it was presented, which resulted in a delayed diagnosis. This underscores the point that uncertainty, precisely because it is ubiquitous in medical practice, must be handled carefully: It can serve as an impetus for further research, but it should never be ignored, nor should it be "eliminated" without the appropriate level of supporting evidence.

4.8. DIAGNOSTIC UNCERTAINTY

It is important to remember that when a patient enters the examination room, the patient and the examining physician enter into a relationship with one another. The patient comes to the physician because the patient has a problem that they hope the physician will be able to address. Thus, the patient exhibits some level of confidence in the physician merely by paying a visit to the clinic. The physician, in turn, by virtue of having medical training and experience, has tools to address the cause of the patient's symptoms. This does not mean that the physician will be able to diagnose, treat, or cure every patient's condition. What it does mean, however, is that a physician, when acting in their proper role, can effectively evaluate a patient and decide either that (1) they are able to diagnose the patient's problem immediately or (2) that further investigation is warranted. Our focus has been on cases of the second type, in which immediate (accurate) diagnosis is not possible. I have argued in this chapter that in these types of cases, the patient's complaints should never be dismissed. Refraining from this kind of dismissal, in addition to its methodological and epistemic virtues, shows respect for the patient by taking the patient at their word. The act of taking the patient at their word shows that the physician is willing to enter into a partnership with the patient and that the physician is willing to listen to the patient, who is, after all, the expert on their own symptoms. As we have seen, if the physician is dismissive of the patient's history, the physician runs the risk of neglecting important pieces of evidence that come from the patient's self-report. Furthermore, as we have seen, a physician who does not consider a patient's complete history is more likely to make poor inferences in the clinical setting. In other words, if the physician is dismissive of the patient's concerns, the physician will not be a good doctor. This is not simply because acting dismissively is both unkind and disrespectful but, rather, because it can result in the physician missing potentially helpful pieces of evidence, and one cannot practice medicine well without taking into account all of the evidence. Finally, it must be recognized that even in the best cases, in which the physician and the patient are engaged in a relationship of mutual respect, sometimes a diagnosis can be made immediately and sometimes it cannot. In some cases, due to practical constraints, investigation might need to be stopped, even before a diagnosis is reached. However, even in cases in which a diagnosis cannot be made (immediately or at all), this situation (a relationship of mutual respect) is preferable to one in which the physician dismisses the patient's concerns.

In this chapter, I have argued that an effective management of diagnostic uncertainty must begin with an ability to recognize and acknowledge it in routine cases in the clinical setting. However, even when diagnostic uncertainty is recognized, this alone is not enough for effective diagnostic practice: Once it is recognized, it must then also be clearly communicated to the patient. If these steps are taken in routine cases, then it will become automatic to do so in even the most complex situations, and diagnostic practice will be the better for it.

Chapter 5

Avoiding Over- and Underdiagnosis

5.1. BACKGROUND

Two potentially harmful diagnostic pitfalls that we have yet to discuss in detail are the problems of overdiagnosis and underdiagnosis. Overdiagnosis has been widely discussed in recent medical literature; however, despite this, precisely what constitutes an instance of "overdiagnosis" is far from agreed upon. Some (Rogers and Mintzker 2016) have argued that the term "refers to diagnosis that does not benefit patients because the diagnosed condition is not a harmful disease in those individuals" (p. 580). Others consider an overdiagnosis to be a diagnosis that "will not lead to an overall benefit to the patient" or that makes "people patients unnecessarily" (Broderson et al. 2018, p. 1). Still others argue that "cases of overdiagnosis are not cases of disease" at all but, rather, "unwarranted labeling of disease" (Hofmann 2017, p. 454).

Following along these lines, I use the term *overdiagnosis* in this chapter to refer to the diagnosis of a patient with a condition that is not currently causing the patient to suffer and will not cause the patient to suffer even if left undiagnosed (and untreated) for the duration of the patient's lifetime. Thus, on this view, the concept of overdiagnosis is not separated from the concept of human suffering.

I reject, on the other hand, definitions of overdiagnosis that equate the term with an "unactionable" diagnosis—which is a diagnosis that does not (or cannot) lead to any sort of clinical action. As discussed previously, there is a common sentiment in clinical medicine that a diagnostic test should not be performed unless it will change what would or could be done for a patient (Sox et al. 2007). For those who argue in this way, "unactionable diagnoses" should be avoided at all costs. They argue that if we cannot do anything about a diagnosis (or do not know what to do), then we should refrain from making the diagnosis at all. Although this is a dominant way of thinking among physicians, not all agree, and some argue that their patients, as a general rule, "have a right to know" what is going to happen to them, even when nothing can be done to change their prognosis. However, on the other hand, there are many cases in which we *could* do something about a condition, even though this would not necessarily be preferable for, and could even be harmful to, the patient. These are cases that count as overdiagnosis, which can in turn lead to overtreatment, something that clearly should be avoided.

On the opposite end of the spectrum from overdiagnosis is the diagnostic pitfall of *underdiagnosis*, which can be understood as the phenomenon of delayed diagnosis, misdiagnosis (incorrect diagnosis), or "missed" diagnosis—that is, not diagnosing the patient at all. Compared to overdiagnosis, the problem of underdiagnosis has received relatively little attention in medical circles. However, it is arguably just as problematic as overdiagnosis and often results in increased suffering for the patient—physically, financially, or both—and therefore it too has both negative pragmatic and ethical implications.

For example, as discussed in previous chapters, significant amounts of time and money (on repeated hospital or clinic visits and/or unnecessary tests and medications) are often wasted in cases of delayed diagnosis, which is a form of clinical underdiagnosis. Thus, the goal in medicine should of course be to avoid both over- and underdiagnosis in clinical practice. In what follows, I argue that this can be done in two ways: by carefully choosing the correct screening and/or diagnostic tests for the given (suspected) condition and then by interpreting the results of those tests in light of the totality of clinical evidence. To understand these two strategies more clearly, it is helpful to consider two examples.

5.2. EXAMPLE 1: WHEN SCREENING LEADS TO UNDERDIAGNOSIS OR OVERDIAGNOSIS: THYROID-STIMULATING HORMONE TESTING AND HYPOTHYROIDISM

Hypothyroidism is a common endocrine disorder that occurs when the thyroid releases too little hormone into the blood. Although no two hypothyroid patients present exactly alike, symptoms of the condition include weight gain or difficulty losing weight, decreased appetite, goiter, dry skin, constipation, depression, yellow tint to the skin, periorbital edema, malabsorption, and slow heart rate. Screening for hypothyroidism generally involves measuring a serum thyroid-stimulating hormone (TSH) level, whereas diagnosis requires a follow-up free thyroxine (FT4) test. TSH is produced by the pituitary gland: When the pituitary is functioning properly, it releases more TSH into the bloodstream when additional thyroid hormone is needed, and it releases less when less is needed. Thus, levels of TSH can be used to indirectly test thyroid function (an elevated TSH suggests hypothyroidism). FT4, on the other hand, is a test that directly measures the amount of available, unbound thyroid hormone in the blood and thus arguably provides a more accurate way to determine thyroid function in a patient. The current guidelines of the American Association of Clinical Endocrinologists recommend TSH as a screening tool for detecting abnormal thyroid function. In general, if a TSH test reveals an elevated level, then the potential diagnosis of hypothyroidism is confirmed by measuring the serum FT4. The problem with this method of screening is that it is well known that not all cases of hypothyroidism present with an elevated TSH. In secondary hypothyroidism, for example, the TSH level is low, and in some cases of clinical hypothyroidism, the TSH is in the normal range. Because a normal TSH result alone proves to be a poor indicator of the body's overall thyroid status (because it does not rule in or out either low or high levels of thyroid hormone in the blood or symptoms in the patient), using this test to screen for hypothyroidism can result in subsequent underdiagnosis of the condition. If the TSH level is within the normal range, and there is no follow-up testing (which is generally the case when the TSH is normal), clinical hypothyroidism may be missed in the patient.

Furthermore, using TSH as a screening test also creates the un-necessary (over)diagnostic category of subclinical hypothyroidism (Skugor 2014). This condition is defined as a normal FT4 with an elevated TSH in an asymptomatic patient. Because the FT4 level is normal in this condition and the patient is asymptomatic, the di-agnostic category of subclinical hypothyroidism is unnecessary. In addition, in many cases it leads to overtreatment because guidelines often suggest initiating thyroid replacement in this subclinical con-dition. If patients were tested with a FT4 assay directly instead of using a TSH test first, then this unnecessary diagnostic category would be eliminated: An asymptomatic patient with a normal FT4 would simply be considered "euthyroid." Furthermore, if FT4 were to be performed directly, as a first step, then the unnecessary costs of performing two tests (a TSH for screening followed by a FT4 to confirm diagnosis when it is elevated) would thereby be avoided. Thus, this example shows that as an important first step toward avoiding both underdiagnosis and overdiagnosis (as well as under- and overtreatment), clinicians need to carefully select both the screening and the diagnostic tests that they will use to inform their decision-making process.

5.3. EXAMPLE 2: MEDICAL IMAGING AND INCIDENTAL FINDINGS

In recent years, there has been a rapid increase in the number of imaging tests performed by clinicians for diagnostic purposes. This is due, at least in part, to the widespread belief that these methods of testing increase diagnostic accuracy. However, as will be demonstrated, the results of these imaging tests—even highly accurate ones—are alone not enough to make accurate diagnoses in the clinical setting. Instead, careful interpretation of these results in light of other supporting evidence is also required. To see this in more detail, consider the following (fictional) case study:

A 20-year-old female presents to the clinic describing intermittent headache, which is sometimes severe enough to cause vomiting, as well as visual disturbance, that started one year prior, shortly after sustaining a concussion. Magnetic resonance imaging (MRI) performed at this time reveals the presence of an arachnoid cyst.

Arachnoid cysts are fluid-filled sacs that can occur either on the arachnoid membrane that covers the brain (intracranial arachnoid cyst) or on the spinal cord. The most common locations for intracranial arachnoid cysts are the middle fossa (near the temporal lobe); the suprasellar region (near the third ventricle); and the posterior fossa, which contains the cerebellum, pons, and medulla oblongata. In many cases, arachnoid cysts do not cause symptoms. However, in cases in which symptoms do occur, headaches, seizures, and abnormal accumulation of excessive cerebrospinal fluid in the brain (hydrocephalus) are common.

A diagnosis of arachnoid cysts is often made incidentally, most commonly during a diagnostic workup for seizures, headaches, or other neurological conditions. In other cases, the diagnosis of an arachnoid cyst may be suspected based on a patient history and a clinical examination, and it may subsequently be confirmed by either computed tomography (CT) or MRI. CT scans and MRIs can thus unexpectedly reveal or, alternatively, confirm the presence of already suspected arachnoid cysts. Of further diagnostic importance is the fact that in most cases, arachnoid cysts are congenital. Less commonly, arachnoid cysts may develop due to head injury, tumor, infection, or brain surgery. Regardless of the cause, these cysts can be either asymptomatic or symptomatic.

Although in the fictional case the patient's symptoms started almost immediately after the concussion, and thus it seems likely that the concussion is their cause, what is not clear in this case is whether or not the patient's symptoms are related in any way to the arachnoid cyst. Notice that this particular uncertainty is unrelated to the accuracy of the MRI. Even if the MRI is an accurate representation of the situation in the patient (i.e., even if the cyst is "really" there and not some sort of imaging artifact), the uncertainty remains because the patient had no baseline MRI prior to the concussion, nor did she receive one at the time the concussion was diagnosed. Thus, it would not be possible for the team to determine whether (1) the concussion caused the arachnoid cyst or (2) the concussion potentially exacerbated a previously present arachnoid cyst. In other words, even if the MRI is accurate in this case, the diagnosis of the patient is still uncertain because it is not clear whether or not her symptoms are due to the presence of the cyst. Yet, the answer to this question matters: If the cyst is causing the symptoms, then it will need to be removed, either by open craniotomy and fenestration or by extracranial shunting. Both of these procedures carry a significant medical risk, but they also both carry a significant potential benefit: If the cyst is the cause of the patient's symptoms, then removing it will relieve the patient of those symptoms. On the other hand, if the presence of the cyst is unrelated to the patient's symptoms, then either of these treatment procedures would be a waste of time and resources and would also be too risky for the patient to undergo.

In this example, we have thus far assumed that the MRI is an accurate representation of the state of affairs in the patient's brain. However, in many cases of medical imaging, additional epistemic uncertainty arises because medical images are not simply photographs:

> In contrast, the format of data from functional neuroimaging experiments is not originally in the format of an image, but rather in terms of data structures that encode numerical values of phase and frequency-dependent signal intensity collected in an abstract framework called "k-space." Visual representations of data in k-space bear no visual resemblance to images of brains. These data are transformed to spatial values of signal intensity with a Fourier transform, resulting in an image that looks roughly brain-like. This analytical transformation doesn't alter the information encoded in the data, and thus may be taken not to introduce any inferential distance, in that it introduces no error or

range of possible causes. However, the radical transformations in format are indication of the indirectness of the technique relative to photography. The fact that these transformations are completely invisible to the consumer of the image implies that neuroimages are not revelatory, and illustrates the inaptness of the imposition of an epistemic framework paradigmatic of photography. (Roskies 2008, p. 25)

What this "inferential distance" means is that

ambiguities and lack of complete data, and physical limitations such as diffraction, field non-uniformity and so on, prevent the image from being an exact representation of what would be seen if the imaged part of the patient were to be exposed to direct vision or drawn by an artist. (Sarvazyan, Lizzi, and Wells 1991, p. 329)

Indirect representation or "inferential distance" and the question of accuracy is not a problem that is specific to medical imaging. In fact, most (if not all) scientific models, whether in physics, biology, chemistry or economics, can be understood as indirect representations of their target systems as well. The question that we most often want to answer with regard to scientific (or medical) models or images is: Do these indirect representations provide good—or at least adequate—explanations of the target systems that they represent? Or, in the medical context specifically, how can medical images, which are incomplete representations, be used to facilitate an accurate diagnosis?

In the philosophy of science literature, attempts to answer the question of how scientific models explain have generally centered on first analyzing the concept of representation because it is usually assumed that scientific models explain because they represent their target systems to some degree of accuracy. But although many philosophers of science agree that scientific representation is important for model explanations, what exactly representation amounts to has been the subject of much debate. Most accounts of scientific representation, however, rest on a common understanding that there is either a formal or an informal relationship of similarity between a model (or image) and the target system that it represents and that this relationship is the basis of the model's/image's representative and explanatory power. Furthermore, in many cases, scientific models or images are thought to explain via comparison cases (Kennedy 2012; Jebeile and Kennedy 2016). Arguably, this is also often the way medical images work in a diagnostic context. That is, when working toward a diagnosis, physicians often mentally compare a medical image with an image of the relevant patient body part reconstructed from "a knowledge base of anatomy, pathology, histology, physical properties of tissues etc." (Sarvazyan et al. 1991, p. 330). If the two images differ, then this information can be used as evidence toward a diagnosis of disease or disorder.

However, because we are of course interested in making correct diagnoses in medicine, one might well ask whether or not the image displayed on the monitor accurately represents the reality in the patient in question (Chhem 2010). This is not a simple question to answer because

the black and white image obtained is conventionally "displayed" as a variation of tissue densities (CT), signal intensities (MRI) or echogenicity (ultrasound). To make this "scientific image" to closer resemble the actual [body part], computer programs enable the manipulations of cross-sectional 2-d images into a volumetric image. This is "post-processing," i.e., processing after the data set was acquired. The result is a "3-d reconstruction" of the 2-d images. (Chhem 2010, p. 12)

In other words, the image is clearly an artificially created one, and we are left with the question, What is "the link between the patient's body part and the image displayed on the monitor" (p. 11)? That is, we are left with the question of when or whether the MRI or CT images in question "provide sufficient information to achieve a diagnosis" (p. 12). The answer to this question is that a medical image alone is never enough for an accurate diagnosis, no matter how accurate a representation it is. Instead, the medical image, because it is a form of indirect observation, must be interpreted, and this requires an appeal to other forms of evidence, such as those derived from the clinical context.

The fictional case study detailed here provides some insight into how to do this. The case is representative of many others like it both because of the diagnostic uncertainty inherent in it and because of the fact that the medical team will be required to act even despite this uncertainty. Diagnostic uncertainty is often present in medical imaging cases such as this one both because medical images, as previously discussed, are indirect representations of what is occurring in the patient and because "advanced imaging studies show tremendous details of pathology. [But] they can also show incidental findings that are of unclear significance" (Hitezman and Cotton 2014, p. 786). What this means, practically speaking, is that although diagnostic images can accurately reveal masses, lesions, and other pathologic structures, these images alone do not a diagnosis make. As discussed in previous chapters, this is true of all diagnostic tests, not just of imaging studies: In order for the result of a diagnostic test to have any significance in the clinical context, that result must be given an interpretation. Again, this is the case independent of the accuracy of the test in question.

In this particular fictional example, there is an extra layer of uncertainty regarding the interpretation of the MRI result because of the lack of a baseline study. In fact, one might wonder whether imaging studies should even be performed in cases such as this if the medical team will question the results of the diagnostic study, no matter what it reveals. The answer to this question is not a simple one, but the short version of the answer is that the diagnostic process in cases such as this is not much different than the process in cases in which baseline studies are available. In both types of case, the diagnosis will depend both on what the imaging study shows and on the clinical context. If the imaging study reveals a dramatic finding, then more weight should be given to the consideration of its diagnostic significance. Similarly, when patient symptoms are severe, even modest imaging findings can be of significant clinical importance.

Perhaps this appeal to clinical evidence for interpreting a diagnostic test seems obvious. However, it is in actuality an implicit critique of the evidence-based medicine (EBM) paradigm. Although the EBM movement has been applauded for moving away from the old style of paternalistic medicine that privileged a physician's clinical experience above all else, it has also been criticized for its overreliance on statistical studies, as well as on diagnostic images and tests. Some have argued against this sort of view that we should instead be pluralists with regard to what counts as medical evidence. For example, Clarke et al. (2014) argue that both statistical and mechanistic evidence are required in order to establish a causal claim (about treatment effectiveness) in medicine. Similarly, I think we can expand upon this view to argue that more than one sort of evidence is also required to establish a causal diagnosis in the clinical setting. Although diagnostic studies, images, and tests are indeed valuable evidence toward a diagnosis, they are only one sort of evidence, not the only sort; case studies, mechanistic reasoning, patient interviews, and even physical examinations should also be counted as evidence toward a diagnosis. Again, this is because even when diagnostic studies provide accurate information, this information is meaningless unless it is given an interpretation in the clinical context. Stanley (2019) makes a similar point:

> Though probabilistic considerations, such as Bayesian estimations of the probability of disease given test results, are important, they are not sufficient for diagnosis selection. If these probabilistic calculations are isolated from careful observation of the particular facts of the clinical case, and if assigned prior probabilities are not tuned to clinical experience and insight, then exclusive consideration of probabilities may lead to misdiagnosis. (p. 439)

Furthermore, this other, non-test-based evidence should not be considered to be weak, lesser, or merely supportive. For instance, as mentioned previously, in more than 80 percent of cases a correct diagnosis can be made on the basis of a patient history alone (Summerton 2008), and, thus if "the history and physical examination are linked properly by the physician's reasoning capabilities, laboratory tests should in large measure be confirmatory" (Campbell and Lynn 1990, p. 37).

If this is the ideal process of diagnosis, what does it mean in practice? Or, to put it in context, how should the medical team in our fictional case proceed? According to our previous definition of overdiagnosis, diagnosing the patient in this case with a symptomatic arachnoid cyst could potentially be wrong in that it could be a *misdiagnosis*, but because the patient is suffering from symptoms, it could not be an *overdiagnosis*. Recall that an overdiagnosis is the diagnosis of a patient with a condition that is not currently causing the patient to suffer and will not cause the patient to suffer if left undiagnosed over the patient's lifetime. Thus, on this definition, an overdiagnosis cannot occur in a symptomatic (suffering) patient. Furthermore, as long as the patient in this case is given a diagnosis of some sort, her diagnosis will not be "missed." But of course more important than classifying the type of diagnosis (or potential diagnostic mistake) in this case, and others like it, is the question of how to proceed under conditions of diagnostic uncertainty. Arguably the best course of action in cases such as this one is to engage the patient in a conversation in which the diagnostic uncertainty as well as the potential treatment options are clearly explained. In other words, diagnostic uncertainty must be communicated to the patient and not hidden. This should be done both because it is epistemically honest and because it is respectful of the patient as an active participant in the health care team. In some diagnostically uncertain cases, the best course of action may be to suspend making a diagnostic judgment. If there is truly insufficient evidence toward a particular diagnosis, and especially if the situation is not urgent, then it might be best to refrain from making a diagnosis until further evidence is gathered or an empirical trial of treatment is conducted. In other words, suspending judgment in a case does not have to result in paralysis or inaction; instead, it can facilitate a treatment trial and/or further investigation.

Importantly, once the diagnostic uncertainty of a case has been communicated to the patient, the patient and the clinician or medical team should then engage in a process of shared decision-making about how to proceed. In the shared decision-making literature, it is widely agreed that patients should be able to make treatment decisions that are in their own best interests—and that sharing the burden of decision-making is best for both patients and practitioners. However, the details of how this process should ideally proceed are often debated. In the case of medical imaging, although many "patients expect, and indeed want, to be informed of any potential laboratory or imaging abnormality that could possibly adversely affect their health, even if the probability that the abnormality could be injurious is highly unlikely" (Hitezman and Cotton 2014, p. 787), in practice, clinicians are not required to give patients all available medical information but only that information which is deemed to be medically relevant. What counts as medically relevant is of course also debated, and some have argued that more information is always better, whereas others argue that too much information can overwhelm and frustrate patients. Here again, I think the best course of action is to approach informed consent and shared decision-making on a case-by-case basis. Patients who want more information are generally entitled to it. On the other hand, patients who want less information are generally entitled to that. The key to ethical and effective communication of epistemic uncertainty in diagnosis is to carefully consider the needs of the individual patient in front of you.

5.4. OVERTREATMENT AND UNDERTREATMENT

Closely related to the diagnostic problems of overdiagnosis and underdiagnosis are the problems of overtreatment and undertreatment. On one end of the spectrum, overtreatment involves treating a patient for a condition that should not be treated, either because the condition does not cause symptoms in the patient or because the treatment for the condition is not effective and could potentially cause the patient harm without benefit. Stegenga (2018) discusses the latter situation and in fact is so concerned about its prevalence in modern medicine that he goes as far as defending what he calls "medical nihilism," which is the thesis that "we should have little confidence in the effectiveness of [most] medical interventions," where "an effective medical intervention is one that improves the health of patients by curing disease or at least treating the symptoms of disease" (p. 23). In fact, he claims not only that we ought to have little confidence in most pharmaceutical interventions but also that we should be very worried about the process by which pharmaceuticals are approved as well as the process by which they are prescribed in clinical practice. On his view, modern medicine is currently operating in such a way that patients throughout the world are being prescribed pharmaceutical interventions, in massive quantities, when there are few reasons to believe that most of these interventions are helpful and in fact many reasons to believe that they might be, on balance, harmful. In my view, this problem is arguably driven, at least in part, by the problem of clinical overdiagnosis.

To begin to see this, consider that Stegenga's (2018) argument is that our "confidence in the effectiveness of a medical intervention can be represented by a conditional probability—the probability that H is true (that the intervention is effective), given the evidence we have: $P(H/E)$" (p. 176). Then, by Bayes' theorem, we have

$$P(H/E) = P(E/H) \times P(H)/P(E)$$

where $P(H)$ is the prior probability that a given intervention will be effective, $P(E/H)$ is the probability of the evidence given that the hypothesis is true, and $P(E)$ is the probability of the evidence. Stegenga then argues that the two terms in the numerator are low, the term in the denominator is high, and thus the probability that a given pharmaceutical intervention will be effective is low. A central component of this argument is that there have been very few "magic bullet" medications in the past, where a magic bullet is defined as an effective pharmaceutical intervention with a specific target. Examples of magic bullets include penicillin for certain bacterial infections and insulin for type 1 diabetes. Because there have been few of these types of pharmaceuticals in the past, the argument goes, we should expect very few of them in the future. Extrapolating from this view, it follows that although we do not need to be skeptical of the effectiveness of *any* new pharmaceutical intervention, we do need to be skeptical about certain classes of pharmaceutical interventions. The pharmaceuticals that we should be skeptical about are the ones that either (1) do not have a specific target or (2) have a specific target but it is not known whether or not modifying that target in turn improves a patient's health. Thus, if Stegenga is correct, we should be skeptical of these kinds of pharmaceutical interventions, precisely because they significantly contribute to the problem of overtreatment.

Notice that with magic bullet interventions, the *cause* of the disease (e.g., proliferation of streptococcus A in strep throat or a deficiency of cortisol in adrenal insufficiency) is well known. Magic bullets, then, are pharmaceutical interventions that intervene effectively on disease conditions that have a simple, known cause. However, many diseases are not causally simple or do not even have a known cause. Thus, any pharmaceutical intervention directed toward curing or ameliorating the symptoms of multicause or unknown-cause diseases is likely to be nonspecific and/or ineffective and thus lead to the overtreatment of patients.

There are several well-known examples of this, including statins as a preventative intervention for heart disease. Heart disease is a major cause of death in developed countries (in the United States, it accounts for roughly one in four deaths) and thus we have good reason to want to develop pharmaceuticals to intervene on this disease process. But because heart disease (and heart attack in particular) does not have one single cause (often not even in an individual patient), it is not easy to develop a pharmaceutical that can effectively intervene on the disease process. Nevertheless, modern medicine has tried to do exactly this by aiming to intervene on one of the potential causes of heart disease: high cholesterol. Although it is known that high cholesterol is often *correlated* with heart disease and that statins do in fact lower cholesterol, it is not known whether this reduction in cholesterol leads to any risk reduction in heart attack rate. Thus, we ought to be skeptical of this type of pharmaceutical intervention.

Another example of a type of intervention we should be skeptical about is the use of selective serotonin reuptake inhibitors (SSRIs) for the treatment of depression. As for heart disease, the causes of depression are multiple and sometimes unknown. Thus, although SSRIs do increase circulating levels of serum serotonin, this does not necessarily alleviate the symptoms of depression in patients who use this intervention. In some cases, SSRIs can make depressive symptoms worse (e.g., the increased risk of suicide that is associated with some SSRIs, such as Prozac).

Statins and SSRIs are examples of drugs that we should be skeptical about because although they have a specific target, it is not known whether or not modifying that target causes an improvement in the specific health conditions that the drugs are intended to treat. Thus, they are drugs for which we should have a low prior probability. One response to this particular problem (of modifying the wrong target or modifying only one target of a multicause disease) by pharmaceutical companies is known as "network pharmacology"

(Hopkins 2008, p. 684), in which the aim is to produce drugs that affect a large number of molecular targets at once. However, not surprisingly, these drugs carry an increased probability of adverse events in patients (Gashaw et al. 2011, pp. 524, 1038).

There are many reasons why we might be concerned about pharmaceutical overtreatment. But what is the alternative? Stegenga (2018) suggests that we should practice "gentle medicine" instead. That is, "we should consume fewer medical interventions, physicians should prescribe fewer interventions and policy-makers should approve fewer interventions" (p. 185). This seems like a reasonable proposal—except of course in medical emergencies or for life-threatening diseases or conditions that cause significant patient suffering. In these cases, both physicians and patients will likely be willing to take on higher risk with regard to potential treatment options.

Undertreatment, on the opposite end of the spectrum from overtreatment, occurs when a patient is not treated at all or is not treated adequately for a condition (diagnosed or not) that is causing the patient to suffer. Undertreatment often accompanies underdiagnosis. For example, untreated or undertreated hypothyroidism can result in serious long-term consequences, including elevated cholesterol, heart rhythm abnormalities, poor immune function, depression, and lethargy. Clearly, then, undertreatment should be avoided just as much as overtreatment.

In some cases, the problems of underdiagnosis/undertreatment occur because the physician mistakenly believes that clinical evidence is weaker or in some other way lesser than the results of diagnostic tests. Thus, the physician might decide not to treat a patient based on negative test results alone, while ignoring relevant clinical data. In the case of hypothyroidism, for example, a physician making this diagnostic mistake might decide that a patient is not hypothyroid and does not require treatment if the TSH level is not elevated, even if clinical symptoms suggest otherwise. However, the opposite is the case with this condition as well as with many others: Although diagnostic testing is clearly useful, it is not the mainstay of the diagnosis.

5.5. CONCLUSION

Undertreatment and overtreatment are major medical issues that are very much intertwined with the diagnostic problems of under- and overdiagnosis: If we do not correctly diagnose a disease (or if we miss it altogether), then there is very little hope that we will be able to treat it effectively. On the other hand, if we diagnose "disease" that does not cause suffering for the patient, then we might end up causing the patient harm from the subsequent overtreatment of the condition. Therefore, in addition to research into the causal basis of diseases, we also need to improve our diagnostic practices by carefully selecting the appropriate screening and/or diagnostic tests as well as by appealing to clinical findings to aid in interpretation of their results.

Furthermore, when (or while) we are not able to identify the cause(s) of a disease and/or are unable to modify the cause(s), medical interventions in such cases should be gentle, not pharmaceutical. If we are unable to develop a "magic bullet" for a condition, then the answer to this problem is not to take the "shotgun" approach. As discussed previously, this type of network pharmacology that promotes multitarget drugs only increases the probability of adverse events in patients. When we are uncertain how to proceed, we should proceed with epistemic humility.

In summary, even when the best test for diagnosing a given condition is utilized, overreliance on diagnostic testing can lead to either overdiagnosis (which can in turn lead to potentially costly or harmful overtreatment) or underdiagnosis (which can lead to repeated and unnecessary testing and clinic visits as well as prolonged patient suffering). Looking to other forms of evidence, aside from that which comes from diagnostic testing, can help reduce these diagnostic errors by facilitating the accurate interpretation of tests conducted in the clinical setting.

Chapter 6

Practicing Diagnostic Justice

6.1. BACKGROUND

The primary focus in the preceding chapters of this book has been on issues related to the diagnosis of individual patients for the purpose of facilitating their clinical care. But as the coronavirus disease 2019 (COVID-19) pandemic has reminded us, individual patients are always part of communities, and this means that in some cases, the diagnosis of individual patients will have ramifications that extend beyond the clinical context of their own treatment to considerations involving the population in which they live. For example, during outbreaks (local or global) of infectious disease, diagnostic testing for both surveillance and subsequent intervention (e.g., containment or mitigation) measures as well as testing for the purpose of individual patient care are simultaneously important. Furthermore, when diagnostic tests become a scarce resource, as was the case in the United States with tests for novel coronavirus at the beginning of the COVID-19 pandemic, the question of how best to allocate these tests arises. Diagnostic situations in which we must weigh societal versus individual benefits and risks can become very complicated, very quickly, and thus require careful thought with regard to deciding why to test, whom to test, and when to test. Thus, in this chapter, I explore the concept of what I call "diagnostic justice" by examining the overlapping categories and the philosophical issues that arise out of diagnostic testing for public health surveillance versus diagnostic testing for clinical care. In particular, I am concerned with the role of the treating physician in making allocation decisions regarding diagnostic tests in the clinical setting.

6.2. DIAGNOSTIC JUSTICE

In order to begin to unpack the concept of diagnostic justice, we must first briefly examine what is meant by the concept of justice more generally. Although a detailed discussion of the concept of justice would fill more than a book (or two or three) on its own, very generally, we might say that justice is what those in a given society, community, or population owe to one another (Scanlon 1998), which is in turn often expressed in terms of the rights and duties of individuals toward one another. Thus, justice is a concept that concerns both individuals and the groups of which they are a part, as well as the relations between these entities. Furthermore, we might say that an action can be labeled "just" or "unjust" for an individual or for the group(s) of which the individual is a member or for both. The specific details, however, of what counts as a just or an unjust action will greatly depend on the context under consideration. In the context of biomedical ethics, for example, much has been written on the idea of justice as fairness, particularly as it relates to the allocation of treatments to patients, especially when these treatments are scarce resources in the community (Beauchamp and Childress 2000; Emanuel, Persad, et al. 2020; Truog, Mitchell, and Daley 2020). Although allocation algorithms for scarce treatments can be very complex, it is generally agreed upon that while competent patients (or their proxies) always have the right to *refuse* a treatment or intervention, they do not have the unmitigated right to *request* or receive these things. This is because although there is no barrier or limit to a patient's *negative* rights to refuse treatments or interventions, a patient's *positive* rights to request and receive these things are in fact limited by several considerations (Brett and McCullough 1986; Simon 2007). For example, one reason that a patient's medical autonomy is limited is because it must be balanced with the physician's (negative) right to refuse to administer a treatment or intervention and, potentially, with the autonomous concerns of other patients. From the clinician's perspective, the patient's autonomy must be balanced with the physician's duty of beneficence (to do good for their patients) as well as with the rights of others in society at large. This means that a physician, even when operating under the principle of beneficence, might be required to refuse to provide an effective, but scarce, treatment to an individual patient in order to allow for the possibility of administering it to someone else who potentially might need it more.

Regarding the concept of *diagnostic justice* specifically, I am concerned in this chapter with the differences between considerations of why to test and whom to test, as these relate to public health, versus considerations of the same as they relate to clinical practice (and thereby to individual patients). In particular, it is important to address the question of how the physician should weigh or rank these potentially competing considerations in the clinical setting when diagnostic testing methods are a scarce resource.

Furthermore, as discussed later, the consideration of diagnostic justice raises some questions that do not generally arise in the discussion of treatment justice: In some cases, that is, it seems that in order for diagnostic justice to be served, a patient's right (to refuse a diagnostic test) must be limited. In order to address this issue, then, we must examine the underlying concern of whose health, exactly, we are talking about when we speak about "public health" and what sacrifices it is acceptable to ask of individuals (in terms of liberty, autonomy, health, or financial resources) within this public in order to achieve it.

6.3. CASE STUDY: COVID-19

COVID-19 is caused by the severe acute respiratory syndrome coronavirus 2 (SARS-CoV-2), which is an enveloped, positive-sense, single-stranded RNA betacoronavirus of the family Coronaviridae. Symptoms of COVID-19 include, but are not limited to, fever, cough, runny nose, shortness of breath, headache, fatigue, sore throat, body aches, and anosmia. According to the Centers for Disease Control and Prevention (CDC), "reported illnesses have ranged from mild symptoms to severe illness and death for confirmed coronavirus disease 2019 (COVID-19) cases" (https://www.cdc.gov/coronavirus/2019-ncov/index.html). Although the infection spreads rapidly and can be severe in some patients, 80 percent of those infected with SARS-CoV-2 have only mild or moderate symptoms (defined as not progressing to pneumonia and not requiring hospital care). COVID-19 is most commonly spread via either close contact (within six feet of an infected person) or by direct contact with the sputum, serum, blood, or respiratory droplets of an infected person.

The first documented case of COVID-19 was detected on December 1, 2019, in Wuhan, China. By December 2020, there were more than 36.7 million documented cases worldwide and more than 1.1 million recorded deaths from the disease.[1] At the

---

1. According to many epidemiologists (who extrapolate from the number of recorded deaths), the number of documented cases likely represents only approximately 10 percent of the number of actual cases worldwide.

beginning of the pandemic, hospital systems throughout the world were quickly overwhelmed by COVID-19 patients, many of whom required intensive care, often in the form of mechanical ventilation. In addition, at the beginning of the pandemic, there were no available vaccines; no proven effective treatments; and very little understanding of transmission, progression, or prognosis of the disease caused by COVID-19.

6.4. DIAGNOSIS VERSUS SURVEILLANCE

Testing for the novel coronavirus includes both DNA and antigen testing for the detection of active infection as well as antibody testing in order to determine past exposure and possible immunity to the virus. Testing for active COVID-19 infection is most often done via polymerase chain reaction (PCR) testing on a nasopharyngeal sample. It works in the following way:

> Samples are taken from places likely to have the virus that causes COVID-19, like the back of the nose or mouth or deep inside the lungs. After a sample is collected, RNA, which is part of the virus particle, is extracted and converted to complementary DNA for testing. The PCR test involves binding sequences on the DNA that only are found in the virus and repeatedly copying everything in between. This process is repeated many times, with doubling of the target region with each cycle. A fluorescent signal is created when amplification occurs, and once the signal reaches a threshold, the test result is considered positive. If no viral sequence is present, amplification will not occur, resulting in a negative result. (Hadaya, Schumm, and Livingston 2020, p. 1981)

The PCR test for COVID-19 infection is considered to be highly accurate (because PCR testing in general has been shown to be so), but currently no data on sensitivity or specificity of the test are available because there is no gold standard for comparison. (Recall from the discussion in Chapter 2 that the evaluation of the accuracy of a diagnostic test requires a comparison measure.[2]) However, early estimates based on similar PCR tests for other diseases put the specificity of the COVID-19 test very high (close to 100 percent, barring laboratory error) but sensitivity only at approximately 70 percent due to the relative frequency of inadequate sampling as well as the disease's variable incubation period (estimated as two to fourteen days). These two things taken together mean that a negative result from a COVID-19 PCR test does not rule out infection in at least 30 percent of cases (Sharfstein, Becker, and Mello 2020). Instead, a negative result suggests no infection, the possibility that the swabbing method missed the virus, or that the virus was not present in the swabbed region (generally the nasal passage), even if it was present elsewhere in the body (e.g., the gastrointestinal tract) at the time of sampling.

Antigen testing, on the other hand, works by detecting fragments of proteins found on or within the virus, also by testing samples collected from nasal swabs. Antigen testing, although rapid, is generally considered to be less accurate than PCR testing and therefore is used less frequently.

It is also worth noting that a positive COVID-19 test result in an asymptomatic or mildly ill patient does not require immediate or urgent medical attention but does require isolation of the patient in order to prevent infection spread. This means that testing

2. The exception to this is test accuracy determination via Bayesian latent class models, which do not require a gold standard for the evaluation of diagnostics (Koustolos et al. 2020).

for SARS-CoV-2 in patients with severe symptoms is generally done in order to facilitate containment/mitigation and, potentially, treatment, whereas testing in asymptomatic, mildly symptomatic, and moderately symptomatic patients is conducted for containment/ mitigation purposes only.

Testing for past infection with COVID-19 is done via serologic antibody titer [immunoglobulin G (IgG) and/or IgM]. Measuring antibody levels in this disease is not generally thought to have much, if any, utility for individual clinical care (antibodies are usually not detectable until at least fourteen to twenty-one days after infection onset, and immunoassays are almost always less accurate than PCR testing). However, measuring antibody levels in a large segment of the population can help determine how much of the population is or was infected, which in turn allows for an estimation of the level of herd immunity present in that population, assuming that naturally derived antibodies provide immunity to the disease. Herd immunity is a form of indirect, population-level protection from infectious disease that results if a sufficiently high proportion of individuals are immune to the disease. This can be achieved in a population via vaccination or naturally when enough people develop immunity after contracting the disease. However, it "should be understood that herd immunity is not the same as biologic (immunologic) immunity; individuals protected only by indirect herd effects remain fully susceptible to infection, should they ever be exposed" (Fine, Eames, and Heymann 2011, p. 914). The required level of herd immunity to stop the spread of a given disease in a given population can be calculated from the basic reproductive number (R_0):

> If immunity (ie, successful vaccination) were delivered at random and if members of a population mixed at random, such that on

average each individual contacted R_0 individuals in a manner sufficient to transmit the infection, then incidence of the infection
would decline if the proportion immune exceeded $[(R_0 - 1)/R_0]$,
or $[1 - (1/R_0)]$. (Fine et al. 2011, p. 912)

Specifically, R_0 is defined as the expected number of secondary
cases produced by a single (typical) infection in a completely susceptible population—that is, before widespread immunity starts to
develop and before any attempt has been made at immunization.
This number can be calculated using the following equation:

$$R_0 = \tau \cdot \bar{c} \cdot d$$

where τ is the transmissibility (i.e., probability of infection given
contact between a susceptible individual and an infected individual), $\bar{c}$ is the average rate of contact between susceptible
and infected individuals, and d is the duration of infectiousness
(Jones 2007).

Because the R_0 for COVID-19 is estimated to be approximately
3, this means that the level of herd immunity required to stop infection spread of the virus would be approximately

$$[3 - 1/3] = .66$$

Although this is clearly a simplified model, in that it assumes, for
instance, homogeneous mixing in a population—which is rarely, if
ever, the case—it has been widely used in epidemiology as a starting
point for predictions concerning the spread of infectious disease
(e.g., see Fine 1993).

6.5. CHALLENGES

Many challenges with the methods of testing for both active COVID-19 infection and past exposure to the virus have arisen in the context of this global pandemic. One of the most significant challenges seems to be due to unclear testing aims. Is the main goal of testing for active COVID-19 to facilitate surveillance followed by public health intervention measures to prevent the spread of the disease in the population at large? If so, this goal was sorely missed, at least in the United States: Much more widespread testing would have been needed to reach it. Instead, in the United States, the CDC both delayed testing for more than a month after it learned of the virus spread in China (Shear et al. 2020) and limited access to testing to those individuals with known exposure, which resulted in making containment of the virus impossible, necessitating "lockdown" measures instead. This is because containment, as was adequately achieved in some countries early in the pandemic, such as South Korea, requires widespread detection of early cases in combination with contact tracing, neither of which were implemented in the United States in either the earlier or the later stages of the pandemic (Sharfstein et al. 2020).

In the early stages of the pandemic in the United States, public health messages about who should be tested and when were inconsistent, changed rapidly, and varied by state and test availability. For example, in Florida, patients were at one point told to try to obtain a test if they had *any* symptoms consistent with COVID-19 or if they were asymptomatic but had known exposure, whereas at another point, shortly after, they were told to only seek testing if they were both critically ill with COVID-like symptoms and older than age 65 years (Florida Department of Health press release, March

2020). The first two announced testing criteria seemed to be surveillance related, whereas the latter two were more obviously related
to clinical care, underscoring the point that there was no clearly ar-
ticulated testing goal in the public setting.

Furthermore, it soon became clear that the number of tests
being conducted in the United States, combined with the lack of
contact tracing, was inadequate for virus containment. By the end
of March 2020, the country had more confirmed cases than any
other country in the world, even though these confirmed cases no
doubt represented only a fraction of the actual number of cases
of the disease. Once it had become clear that testing for containment purposes had failed, the question then shifted to whether or
not testing for active COVID-19 had any utility for clinical care.
Clinicians began to ask whether or not it is important (for clinical
care) to test those admitted to the intensive care unit for respiratory distress for COVID-19 and, in particular, whether or not the
results of the test would change either their treatment options or
outcomes in any favorable way (Zagury-Orly and Schwartzstein
2020). In other words, at this point the question became whether or
not the test for active COVID-19 had any clinical effectiveness. In
Chapter 3, it was noted that a clinically effective diagnostic test must
not only be accurate but also, in some way, lead to a measurable improvement in the patient's health outcome. In general, as mentioned
previously, diagnostic testing is conducted to facilitate treatment
of individual patients. However, in the case of COVID-19, which
at the time of this writing has no adequately tested or established
method of treatment, it is unclear whether testing for the virus in
patients with symptoms consistent with it makes any difference in
their overall health outcomes.

A positive COVID-19 test in an admitted patient can, however, serve to protect health care workers as well as other patients:

Patients who test positive can be isolated from other patients, and health care workers can be better prepared to take anti-infection precautions when interacting with these patients. However, it is unlikely that a positive test result would have a direct impact on most of the treatment measures to be potentially undertaken in a critically symptomatic patient. Instead, treatment decisions for these patients, which might include intravenous fluids, mechanical ventilation, or high-flow oxygen, would need to be made based on the clinical presentation of the patient, at least until a proven effective COVID-19-specific treatment is found.

An exception to this would be empirical treatment trials in patients who test positive for COVID-19. In this case, it would be important to know that the disease was indeed COVID-19, rather than something else with similar symptoms, in order to reliably evaluate potential treatment effectiveness. To date, there are sixty-four (Gordon et al. 2020) currently in-use drugs that exhibit potential mechanisms of action against SARS-CoV-2. Although full-scale randomized controlled trials are currently underway for many of them, because these often take twelve to eighteen months to complete, clinicians in many hospitals throughout the world are conducting their own small-scale observational studies of drugs such as hydroxychloroquine and remdesivir for the treatment of active COVID-19.

In terms of antibody testing for COVID-19, several interesting questions have also arisen during the pandemic. Aside from the usual concerns about testing accuracy, it is not currently known whether elevated titers of IgG to the virus are protective partially or completely against subsequent infection, or for how long. Although we know that past exposure to most other viral infections often does confer immunity, at least temporarily, this is not always the case. For example, a second infection with the dengue virus is often far worse, clinically, than the first. This seems to be due to the fact that "for dengue viruses 1 to 4 (DENV1–4), a specific range of antibody titer has been shown to enhance viral replication" (Katzelnick et al. 2017, p. 930). With dengue, high levels of antibodies protect against subsequent infection, but as these levels begin to decline over time, there is a sort of "anti-sweet spot" level of antibody that enables the virus to replicate in the host more quickly, causing more severe symptoms in the patient than when no antibodies are present.

Because it was not known how antibody levels interact with the SARS-CoV-2 virus in terms of preventing subsequent infection, or for how long, in April 2020 the World Health Organization issued a statement urging governments not to rely on data from antibody testing to relax social distancing guidelines.

6.6. ANALYSIS

The question of how to allocate diagnostic tests when they are a scarce societal resource can be broken down into two subquestions. In order to effectively, and justly, allocate diagnostic tests, we must answer the following:

Why should we test?
Who should we test?

In order to answer the first question, we must first recall that there are at least three potential reasons to conduct diagnostic testing: (1) surveillance plus subsequent intervention measures at the population level, (2) individual diagnosis followed by treatment measures in the clinical context, and (3) research purposes (including case study analyses and empirical trials) to facilitate effective clinical care for future patients. This means that the answer to the question of why to test could be any of these three reasons or some combination thereof.

The answer to the second question will depend, in large measure, on the answer to the first question. If the purpose of the testing is for surveillance plus intervention—for example, in the context of an infectious disease such as COVID-19—then tests should be administered as widely as possible to anyone who is considered to be potentially contagious (which could, in principle, be the entire population), whether they are symptomatic or not. On the other hand, if the purpose of the diagnostic testing is to facilitate the best possible clinical care for (currently) ill individuals, then tests should be given to symptomatic patients for whom the test result would be likely to change the course of their clinical care (in terms of either treatment or supportive measures). Finally, if the purpose of the testing is to facilitate either randomized or empirical trials to aid in the effective treatment of individuals who will become ill in the future, then testing should be conducted on symptomatic patients even when it is *not known* whether or not the test results would change the course of their clinical care in any significant way. This epistemic requirement that it not be known ahead of time whether or not the treatment is effective is known as the principle of equipoise (Freedman 1987). According to Freedman, equipoise is the state of genuine uncertainty within the expert medical community on the best treatment for a condition. Thus, it is a state that exists when some physicians favor one treatment (or expect it to work) while other clinicians favor another (or do not expect the one being tested to work). The idea is that this epistemic principle should be adhered to because if it is already known prior to the trial that the treatment works, then running the trial is a waste of time and financial resources, whereas if it is already known prior to the trial that the treatment does not work, then the trial participants will be put at risk for no reason.

Sometimes, as certainly seems to be the case in the context of the COVID-19 pandemic, there is good reason to test for the purposes of both surveillance and individual diagnosis. However, if there are not enough tests in order to achieve both goals simultaneously, then these reasons for testing must be ranked. How, then, do we rank the individual versus societal benefits of diagnostic testing in cases such as this? In order to do that, we have to ask, What is the goal of testing for surveillance and mitigation measures? Is the goal to minimize the number of deaths in the population? If so, then we have to model and, as best we can, project whether prevention of disease or treatment of disease would be likely to be more effective in reaching this goal. In the case of COVID-19, the answer to this question is clear: Because there is no established effective treatment for the condition, prevention is the more desirable measure to take. Thus, the goal of testing should be surveillance in addition to mitigation measures in order to halt the proliferation of the disease and thereby prevent as many deaths as possible. As discussed previously, this goal was not reached in the United States. Thus, at that point, the goal of COVID-19 testing shifted to include both individual diagnosis and research purposes. However, this of course only exacerbated the problem of test scarcity because it expanded the reasons for testing from one to three.

To add to the complication, at this point, antibody tests were also introduced. What is the reason for conducting these tests? It is clear that the reason cannot be either individual diagnosis or research purposes, because antibodies to COVID-19 usually only begin to develop fourteen to twenty-one days after symptom onset, which would very likely be too late for either effective clinical care or empirical research. Could the reason potentially be surveillance plus subsequent intervention measures at the population level? As mentioned previously, the idea behind antibody testing during an infectious disease pandemic is that it can give some indication of how many people in the population have contracted the disease and thus how close the population is to achieving herd immunity. However, this information alone does not necessarily further the end of containing the disease or of mitigating its effects because it does not allow for a determination of who is or is not contagious, unless it can be determined that once antibodies have been detected, the period of infectiousness has passed. At least at the time of this writing (December 2020), it was not clear what the goal of antibody testing in the COVID-19 pandemic was supposed to be. However, this was not as problematic as the issues with tests for active infection because there was not as severe a shortage of antibody tests.

One important issue that we have yet to address is the question of when, if ever, it is permissible to *require* diagnostic testing in a population. The idea behind requiring testing is that it would further the end of testing for surveillance plus mitigation or containment measures: The more people who are tested, the more likely it is that the disease will be successfully contained, especially if those in the population who test positive for active infection can be effectively isolated from others. In the context of justice in treatment allocation, it was previously noted that, in general, there are no restrictions on a competent adult patient's right to refuse a treatment measure or intervention. However, this is not as clearly the case with regard to diagnostic testing for surveillance purposes. As with vaccines, diagnostic testing for an infectious disease might be done not solely for the benefit of the individual being tested but also to protect others in the society of which the infected person is a part.

Thus, the answer to the question of whether it is sometimes, always, or never acceptable to force individuals to be tested will depend on how one ranks the good of the individual versus the good of the community with regard to *containment/mitigation measures specifically*. As discussed previously, diagnosis is the very starting point of modern medicine, and without an accurate diagnosis, any ensuing treatment or intervention measures or prognostic predictions will likely fail. But when we speak of the "good of the individual versus the good of the community," in the context of diagnostic surveillance, whose good, or whose health, exactly, are we talking about? One might wonder here why, because communities are composed of individuals, it is not the case that acting in the best interest of each individual in the society will in turn result in furthering the best interest of the community at large. The somewhat obvious answer is that what is in the best interest of one person in a society might not be in the best interest of someone else in that same society. If you and I both become ill with bacterial sepsis and there is only enough antibiotic treatment for one of us, then it is in my best interest that you not get the antibiotic and that I do, whereas the reverse is true for you.

The same is potentially true for scarce diagnostic tests. If, for instance, a future requirement (for insurance or, possibly, standard-of-care reasons) for treatment for COVID-19 is a positive DNA test, if you and I both present with identical symptoms that are consistent with this viral disease but there is only one test available, then it is in my best interest to get the test while you do not. The critical question for the clinician, then, is how to weight societal considerations versus considerations of individual patient care. My proposal for answering this question is that when acting in the role of physician, the clinician must be primarily concerned with the good of the patient that is in front of them. To understand why, imagine the opposite sort of scenario. Imagine that you end up in the emergency department of your local hospital with a diagnosis of sepsis. The treatment for this condition is intravenous antibiotic therapy, generally with two or three agents (Schmidt and Mandel 2020). But suppose that the attending physician in this case decides not to treat you because she is aware that the more often any given antibiotic is prescribed, the more likely it is that bacteria in the community will develop resistance to it. So, she decides not to treat you in order to preserve the antibiotics' effectiveness. Intuitively, most of us would agree that there is something wrong with this physician's decision. What is wrong in this hypothetical case is that the physician has misunderstood the purpose of their role. That is, the role of a physician, and the ethical code by which the physician must abide, differs from that of a medical researcher (Lasagna 1968). The physician must be primarily concerned with the patient as an individual, whereas the researcher is, and should be, primarily concerned with acquiring new, generalizable knowledge that will facilitate health outcomes in the population at large. These two aims of medical practice and medical research are equally important, of course; however, sometimes the two are in tension, and this tension is not something that is likely to disappear any time soon. But what the individual physician must focus on, in the context of clinical care, is the patient whom the physician is treating at that given time: This should take priority over societal considerations.

6.7. CONCLUSION

The purpose of diagnostic testing can be either for the promotion of public health (via either prevention strategies or research studies) or for facilitating the clinical care of individual patients.

When diagnostic tests are scarce, we might be forced to rank these, at times, competing purposes. When doing so, many considerations come into play, including the question of the end goal of the testing being performed, whether that is for prevention, research, or treatment. However, when a clinician is acting in the role of a physician, the clinician's primary responsibility is to the individual patient who is being treated and not to the general public at large. Thus, for the physician, testing (and treatment) allocations should be made, in the first instance, on the basis of the needs of the individual patient, and societal concerns should be secondary in the diagnostic decision-making process. For a medical researcher, on the other hand, the priority is reversed: When acquisition of knowledge is the primary goal, then considerations of individual patients and their care will necessarily be secondary. However, because the practice of medicine always concerns the health of individual people, the goal is never knowledge acquisition alone, but always its application.

Conclusion

The process of clinical diagnosis—from establishing the patient–physician relationship to gathering evidence, to performing, evaluating, interpreting, and allocating diagnostic tests, to settling upon a working explanation for the patient's condition and pursuing a treatment plan, all the while avoiding the pitfalls of both overdiagnosis and underdiagnosis—is arguably the cornerstone of all modern medicine. Via the discussion in this book, I hope I have shown that this process, even in what might be considered to be ordinary or routine cases, is complex, fascinating, multifaceted, and involves considerations of logic, evidence, ethics, probability, and economics. Thus, the process of clinical diagnosis is about far more than just basic science. Here, as in all areas of medical practice, ethics is inextricably intertwined with evidence: Becoming a good diagnostician requires not only an understanding of probability theory and statistical analysis but also learning to listen to your patients, learning how to interpret the results of diagnostic tests by taking into account clinical considerations, learning how to manage and communicate diagnostic uncertainty in the clinical setting, understanding the potential reasons to conduct diagnostic tests or not, and being concerned with issues of diagnostic justice while keeping in mind the concerns of the actual patient who is in front of you.

CONCLUSION

The diagnostic process is not an easy one to master, in part because it requires not only brilliance on the part of the physician but also humility, empathy, and care for the patient. However, it is a skill that can be learned, and improved, over time. Doing so has the potential to bring great reward: When the process of clinical diagnosis is practiced well, it sets the stage for more effective treatments, better clinical outcomes, and greater patient and physician satisfaction. Thus, it is well worth studying and practicing. I hope that this book has motivated you to continue to do so.

REFERENCES

Abdel-Motleb, M. 2012. "The Neuropsychiatric Aspect of Addison's Disease." *Innovations in Clinical Neuroscience* 9: 34–36.

Alla, V., N. Natarajan, M. Kaushik, R. Warrier, and C. K. Nair. 2010. "Paget–Schroetter Syndrome: Review of Pathogenesis and Treatment of Effort Thrombosis." *Western Journal of Emergency Medicine* 11(4): 358–62.

Atkinson, P. 1984. "Training for Certainty." *Social Science and Medicine* 19(9): 949–56.

Barrows, H., and G. Pickell. 1991. *Developing Clinical Problem Solving Skills.* New York: Norton.

Beauchamp, T., and J. Childress. 2000. *Principles of Biomedical Ethics.* Oxford, UK: Oxford University Press.

Beckman, H. B., and R. M. Frankel. 1984. "The Effect of Physician Behavior on the Collection of Data." *Annals of Internal Medicine* 101(5): 692–96.

Berner, E. S., and M. L. Graber. 2008. "Overconfidence as a Cause of Diagnostic Error in Medicine." *American Journal of Medicine* 121(5 Suppl.): S2–S23.

Bensenor, I., R. Olmos, and P. Lotufo. 2012. "Hypothyroidism in the elderly: diagnosis and management." *Clinical Interventions in Aging* 7: 97–111.

Bluhm, R. 2013. "Physiological Mechanisms and Epidemiological Research." *Journal of Evaluation in Clinical Practice* 19: 422–26.

Boorse, C. 2011. "Concepts of Health and Disease." In *Philosophy of Medicine,* edited by F. Gifford, Vol. 16, 13–64. New York: Elsevier.

Bossuyt, P., J. Lijmer, and B. Mol. 2000. "Randomized Comparisons of Medical Tests: Sometimes Invalid, Not Always Efficient." *Lancet* 356: 1844–46.

Bossuyt, P., and K. McCaffery. 2009. "Additional Patient Outcomes and Pathways in Evaluations of Testing." *Medical Decision Making* 29(5): E30–E38.

Botti, S., and S. S. Iyengar. 2004. "The Psychological Pleasure and Pain of Choosing at the Cost of Subsequent Satisfaction." *Journal of Personal Social Psychology* 87(3): 312–26.

Braithwaite, R. S. 2013. "EBM's Six Most Dangerous Words." *JAMA* 310(20): 2149–50. doi:10.1001/jama.2013.281996.

Brett, A. S., and L. McCullough. 1986. "When Patients Request Specific Interventions." *New England Journal of Medicine* 315: 1347–51.

Brett, A. S., and C. Powell. 2011. "Approach to Laboratory Testing and Imaging in Aging." In *Case-Based Geriatrics: A Global Approach*, edited by V. A. Hirth, D. Wieland, and M. Dever-Bumba, 14–21. New York: McGraw-Hill.

Broderson, J., L. M. Schwartz, C. Heneghan, J. W. O'Sullivan, J. K. Aronson, and S. Woloshin. 2018. "Overdiagnosis: What It Is and What It Isn't." *BMJ* 23: 1–3.

Brozek, J. L., E. Akl, and R. Jaeschke. 2009. "The GRADE Approach to Grading Quality of Evidence about Diagnostic Tests and Strategies." *Allergy* 64: 1109–16.

Campbell, E., Jr., and C. Lynn. 1990. "The Physical Examination." In *Clinical Methods: The History, Physical, and Laboratory Examinations*, edited by H. K. Walker, W. D. Hall, and J. W. Hurst, 3rd ed. Boston: Butterworths.

Centers for Disease Control and Prevention. 2020. "Lyme Disease." Retrieved from http://www.cdc.gov/lyme

Chhem, R. 2010. "Medical Image: Imaging or Imagining?" In *Medical Imaging and Philosophy*, edited by H. Fangerau, R. Chhem, I. Muller, and S.-C. Wang. Stuttgart, Germany: Franz Steiner Verlag.

Clarke, B., D. Gillies, P. Illari, F. Russo, and J. Williamson. 2014. "Mechanisms and the Evidence Hierarchy." *Topoi* 33(2): 339–60.

Cournoyea, M., and A. Kennedy. 2014. "Causal Explanatory Pluralism and Medically Unexplained Physical Symptoms." *Journal of Evaluation in Clinical Practice* 20(6): 928–33.

Coon, E., R. A. Quinonez, V. A. Moyer, and A. R. Schroeder. 2014. "Overdiagnosis: how our compulsion for diagnosis may be harming our children." *Pediatrics* 134: 5.

Croce, M. 2018. "Epistemic Paternalism and the Service Conception of Epistemic Authority." *Metaphilosophy* 49(3).

Croskerry, P., and G. Norman. 2008. "Overconfidence in Clinical Decision Making." *American Journal of Medicine* 121(5 Suppl.): S24–S29.

di Ruffano, L. F., J. Dinnes, A. J. Sitch, C. Hyde, and J. J. Deeks. 2017. "Test-Treatment RCTs Are Susceptible to Bias: A Review of the Methodological Quality of Randomized Trials That Evaluate Diagnostic Tests." *BMC Medical Research Methodology* 17: 35.

Dong, B. 2000. "How medications affect thyroid function." *Western Journal of Medicine* 172(2): 102–6.

Djulbegovic, B., I. Hozo, and S. Greenland. 2011. "Uncertainty in Clinical Medicine." In *Philosophy of Medicine*, edited by F. Gifford, 299–356. Oxford, UK: North Holland.

Dorin, R. I., C. R. Qualls, and L. M. Crapo. 2003. "Diagnosis of Adrenal Insufficiency." *Annals of Internal Medicine* 139: 194–204.

Douglas, H. 2008. "The Role of Values in Expert Reasoning." *Public Affairs Quarterly* 22(1): 1–18.

Elliott, K. C., and D. Willmes. 2013. "Cognitive Attitudes and Values in Science." *Philosophy of Science* 80(5): 807–17.

Emanuel, E. J., G. Persad, R. Upshur, B. Thome, M. Parker, A. Glickman, C. Zhang, et al. 2020. "Fair Allocation of Scarce Medical Resources in the Time of Covid-19." New England Journal of Medicine 382: 2049–55.

Emanuel, E. J., D. Wendler, and C. Grady 2000. "What Makes Clinical Research Ethical?" *JAMA* 283(20): 2701–11.

Emanuel, E., and L. Emanuel. 1992. Four Models of the Physician-Patient Relationship. *JAMA* 267(16): 2221–6.

Engelhardt, T. 1975. In *Evaluation and Explanation in the Biomedical Sciences*, edited by H. T. Engelhardt and S. F. Spicker, Vol. 1. Dordrecht, the Netherlands: Springer.

Evidence Based Medicine Working Group. 1992. "Evidence-Based Medicine: A New Approach to Teaching the Practice of Medicine." *Journal of the American Medical Association* 268(17): 2420–25.

Fine, P. 1993. "Herd Immunity: History, Theory, Practice." *Epidemiologic Reviews* 15: 265–302.

Fine, P., K. Eames, and D. L. Heymann. 2011. " 'Herd Immunity': A Rough Guide." *Clinical Infectious Diseases* 52(7): 911–16.

Fox, R. C. 1957. "Training for Uncertainty." In *The Student–Physician: Introductory Studies in the Sociology of Medical Education*, edited by R. K. Merton, G. Reader, and P. L. Kendall, 207–41. Cambridge, MA: Harvard University Press.

Freedman, B. 1987. "Equipoise and the Ethics of Clinical Research." *New England Journal of Medicine* 317: 141–45.

Gashaw, I., P. Ellinghaus, A. Sommer, and K. Asadullah. 2011. "What Makes a Good Drug Target?" *Drug Discovery Today* 16(23–24): 1037–43.

Goldenberg, M. 2013. "How Can Feminist Theories of Evidence Assist Clinical Reasoning and Decisionmaking?" *Social Epistemology* 29: 3–30.

Goldenberg, M. 2016. "More Than Patient-Centered Care, Patient Expertise." *BMJ* 354.

Gordon, D E., G. M. Jang, M. Bouhaddou, J. Xu, K. Obernier, M. J. O'Meara, J. Z. Guo, et al. 2020. "A SARS–CoV-2–Human Protein–Protein Interaction Map Reveals Drug Targets and Potential Drug Repurposing." Retrieved from https://doi.org/10.1101/2020.03.22.002386

Grove, W., D. H. Zald, B. S. Lebow, B. E. Snitz, and B. Nelson. 2000. "Clinical vs. Mechanical Prediction: A meta-analysis." *Psychological Assessment* 12(1): 19–30.

Guram, D. L. 2011. "The Art of Diagnosis." *South Carolina Medicine* [Online]. Retrieved from http://www.med.sc.edu/SC%20Medicine_final.pdf

REFERENCES

Hadaya, J., M. Schumm, and E. Livingston. 2020. "Testing Individuals for Coronavirus 2019 (COVID-19)." *JAMA* 323(19): 1981. doi:10.1001/jama.2020.5388

Hiroi, N., A. Yoshihara, M. Sue, G. Yoshino, and M. Higa. 2010. "Central Adrenal Insufficiency and Diabetes Insipidus Misdiagnosed as Severe Depression." *Clinical Medicine Insights Case Reports* 3: 55–58.

Hitezman, N., and C. Cotton. 2014. "Incidentalomas: Initial Management." *American Family Physician* 90: 784–89.

Hofmann, B. 2016. "Incidental Findings of Uncertain Significance: To Know or Not to Know—That Is Not the Question." *BMC Medical Ethics* 17: 13.

Hofmann, B. 2017. "The Overdiagnosis of What? On the Relationship Between the Concepts of Overdiagnosis, Disease, and Diagnosis." *Medicine, Health Care, and Philosophy* 20: 453–64.

Hopkins, A. 2008. "Network Pharmacology: The Next Paradigm in Drug Discovery." *Nature Chemical Biology* 4(11): 682–90.

Howick, J. 2011. *The Philosophy of Evidence-Based Medicine.* Oxford, UK: Wiley-Blackwell.

Iwata, M., G. Hazama, Y. Shirayama, T. Ueta, S. Yoshioka, and R. Kawahara. 2004. "A Case of Addison's Disease Presented with Depression as a First Symptom." *Seishin Shinkeigaku Zasshi* 106: 1110–16.

Jebeile, J., and A. Kennedy 2016. "Explaining with Models: The Role of Idealizations." *International Studies in the Philosophy of Science* 29(4): 383–92.

Jones, J. 2007. "Notes on R_0." Retrieved from https://web.stanford.edu/~jhj1/teachingdocs/Jones-on-R0.pdf

Katz, U., A. Achiron, Y. Sherer, and Y. Shoenfeld. 2007. "Safety of Intravenous Immunoglobulin Therapy." *Autoimmunity Reviews* 6(4): 257–59.

Katzelnick, L. C., L. Gresh, M. E. Halloran, J. C. Mercado, G. Kuan, A. Gordon, A. Balmaseda, and E. Harris. 2017. "Antibody-Dependent Enhancement of Severe Dengue Disease in Humans." *Science* 358(6365): 929–32.

Kennedy, A. G. 2012. "A Non Representationalist View of Model Explanation." Studies in History and Philosophy of Science 43(2): 326–32.

Kennedy, A. G. 2013. "Differential Diagnosis and the Suspension of Judgment." *Journal of Medicine and Philosophy* 38(5): 487–500.

Kennedy, A. G., and S. Malanowski. 2018. "Mechanistic Reasoning and Informed Consent." *Bioethics* 33(1): 162–68.

Knotternus, J. A., and F. Buntinx. 2008. *The Evidence Base of Clinical Diagnosis.* Oxford, UK: Wiley-Blackwell.

Koustoulos, P., P. Eusebi, and S. Hartnack. 2020. "Diagnostic Accuracy Estimates for COVID-19 RT-PCR and Lateral Flow Immunoassay Tests with Bayesian Latent Class Models." Retrieved from https://www.researchsquare.com/article/rs-33243/v1

Kullberg, B. J., H. D. Vrijmoeth, F. van de Schoor, and W. J. Hovius. 2020. "Lyme Borreliosis: Diagnosis and Management." *BMJ* 369: m1041.

Lasagna, L. 1968. "Some Ethical Problems in Clinical Investigation." *SA Medical Journal* 42(1): 2–5.

Lijmer, J., and Bossuyt, P. 2009. "Various randomized designs can be used to evaluate medical tests." *Journal of Clinical Epidemiology* 62: 364–73.

Likes, K., D. Rochlin, S. Nazarian, M. Streiff, and J. Freislag. 2013. "Females with Subclavian Vein Thrombosis May Have an Increased Risk of Hypercoagulability." *JAMA Surgery* 148(1): 44–49.

Lovas, K., and E. S. Husebye. 2002. "High Prevalence and Increasing Incidence of Addison's Disease in Western Norway." *Clinical Endocrinology* 56: 787–91.

Martinez, M. 2012. "Managing Scientific Uncertainty in Medical Decision Making: The Case of the Advisory Committee on Immunization Practices." *Journal of Medicine and Philosophy* 37: 6–27.

Marvel, K., R. M. Epstein, K. Flowers, and H. B. Beckman. 1999. "Soliciting the Patient's Agenda—Have We Improved?" *JAMA* 281(3): 283–87.

Mrazek, V., and P. Bartunek. 1999. "Lyme Borreliosis." *Casopís lékařů českých* 138: 329–32.

Musschenga, B. 2019. "Is There a Problem with False Hope?" *Journal of Medicine and Philosophy* 44: 423–41.

Racine, E., J. Aspler, C. Forlini, and J. A. Chandler. 2017. "Contextualized Autonomy and Liberalism: Broadening the Lenses on Complementary and Alternative Medicines in Preclinical Alzheimer's Disease." *Kennedy Institute of Ethics Journal* 27(1): 1–41.

Rencic, J., R. L. Trowbridge, Jr., M. Fagan, K. Szauter, and S. Durning. 2017. "Clinical Reasoning Education at US Medical Schools: Results from a National Survey of Internal Medicine Clerkship Directors." *Journal of General Internal Medicine* 32(11): 1242–46.

Reyna, V. 2008. "A Theory of Medical Decision Making and Health: Fuzzy Trace Theory." *Medical Decision Making* 28(6): 850–65.

Rodger, M., T. Ramsay, and D. Fergusson. 2012. "Diagnostic Randomized Controlled Trials: The Final Frontier." *Trials* 13: 137.

Rogers, W., and Y. Mintzker. 2016. "Getting Clearer on Overdiagnosis." *Journal of Evaluation in Clinical Practice* 22: 580–87.

Rorat, M., E. Kuchar, L. Szenborn, and K. Małyszczak. 2010. "Growing Borreliosis Anxiety and Its Reasons." *Psychiatria Polska* 44: 895–904.

Roskies, A. 2008. "Neuroimaging and Inferential Distance." *Neuroethics* 1: 19–30.

Sackett, D. 1996. "Evidence based medicine. What it is and what it isn't." *BMJ* 312: 71–2.

Sackett, D. L., S. E. Straus, W. S. Richardson, W. Rosenberg, and R. B. Haynes. 2000. *Evidence-Based Medicine: How to Practice and Teach EBM.* Edinburgh, UK: Churchill-Livingstone.

Sadegh-Zadeh, K. 2011. "The Logic of Diagnosis." In *Handbook of Philosophy of Science, Vol. 16: Philosophy of Medicine*, edited by F. Gifford, 357–424. New York: Elsevier.

REFERENCES

Sadler, J. 2005. *Values and Psychiatric Diagnosis.* Oxford University Press.

Sarvazyan, A. P., F. L. Lizzi, and P. N. Wells. 1991. "A New Philosophy of Medical Imaging." *Medical Hypotheses* 36(4): 327–35.

Schwab, A. 2012. "Epistemic Humility and Medical Practice: Translating Epistemic Categories into Ethical Obligations." *Journal of Medicine and Philosophy* 37: 28–48.

Scanlon, T. M., 1998. *What We Owe to Each Other.* Cambridge, MA: Harvard University Press.

Schmidt, G., and J. Mandel. 2020. "Evaluation and Management of Suspected Sepsis and Septic Shock in Adults." Retrieved from https://www.uptodate.com/contents/evaluation-and-management-of-suspected-sepsis-and-septic-shock-in-adults

Shahar, E. 1997. "A Popperian Perspective on the Term 'Evidence-Based Medicine.'" *Journal of Evaluation in Clinical Practice* 3(2): 109–16.

Sharfstein, J., S. J. Becker, and M. M. Mello. 2020. "Diagnostic Testing for the Novel Coronavirus." *JAMA* 323(15): 1437–38. doi:10.1001/jama.2020.3864

Shear, M., D., A. Goodnough, S. Kaplan, S. Fink, K. Thomas, and N. Weiland. 2020. "The Lost Month: How a Failure to Test Blinded the U.S. to Covid-19." *The New York Times.* Retrieved from https://www.nytimes.com/2020/03/28/us/testing-coronavirus-pandemic.html?campaign_id=9&emc=edit_nn_20200329&instance_id=17169&nl=morningbriefing&regi_id=115480088&segment_id=23230&te=1&user_id=f2db0943d1a7193b5672a1bad6da4481

Simon, J. R. 2007. "Refusal of Care: The Physician–Patient Relationship and Decisionmaking Capacity." *Annals of Emergency Medicine* 50(4): 456–61.

Simpkin, A. L., and R. M. Schwartzstein. 2016. "Tolerating Uncertainty: The Next Medical Revolution?" *New England Journal of Medicine* 375: 1713–15.

Simpkin, A. L., J. M. Vyas, and K. A. Armstron. 2017. "Diagnostic Reasoning: An Endangered Competency in Internal Medicine Training." *Annals of Internal Medicine* 167: 507–9.

Skugor M. 2014. "Hypothyroidism and Hyperthyroidism." Cleveland Clinic Foundation Center for Continuing Education. Retrieved from http://www.clevelandclinicmeded.com/medicalpubs/diseasemanagement/endocrinology/hypothyroidism-and-hyperthyroidism/#cetextbox3

Smith, R., and D. Francesca. 2007. "Classification and Diagnosis of Patients with Medically Unexplained Symptoms." *Journal of General Internal Medicine* 22(5): 685–91.

Sox, H., M. A. Blatt, M. C. Higgins, and K. I. Marton. 2007. *Medical Decision Making.* Philadelphia, PA: American College of Physicians.

Stanley, D. 2019. "The Logic of Medical Diagnosis: Generating and Selecting Hypotheses." *Topoi* 38: 437–46.

Stanley, D., and D. Campos. 2013. "The Logic of Medical Diagnosis." *Perspectives in Biology and Medicine* 56(2): 300–15.

Stegenga, J. 2018. *Medical Nihilism*. Oxford University Press.

Stricker, R. B. 2007. "Counterpoint: Long-Term Antibiotic Therapy Improves Persistent Symptoms Associated with Lyme Disease." *Clinical Infectious Diseases* 45: 149–57.

Summerton, N. 2008. "The Medical History as a Diagnostic Technology." *British Journal of General Practice* 58(549): 273–76.

Tekin, Ş. 2016. "Are Mental Disorders Natural Kinds? A Plea for a New Approach to Intervention in Psychiatry." *Philosophy, Psychiatry, and Psychology* 23(2): 147–63.

Truog, R. D., C. Mitchell, and G. Q. Daley. 2020. "The Toughest Triage—Allocating Ventilators in a Pandemic." *New England Journal of Medicine* 382: 1973–75

Upshur, R. E. 2000. "Seven Characteristics of Medical Evidence." *Journal of Evaluation in Clinical Practice* 6(2): 93–97.

Upshur, R. E. 2005. "Looking for Rules in a World of Exceptions: Reflections on Evidence-Based Practice." *Perspectives in Biology and Medicine* 48: 477–89.

Upshur, R., and B. Chin-Yee. 2017. "Clinical Judgment." In *The Routledge Companion to Philosophy of Medicine*, edited by M. Solomon, J. Simon, and H. Kincaid, 363–370. New York: Routledge.

Urschel, H., and A. Patel. 2008. "Surgery Remains the Most Effective Treatment for Paget–Schroetter Syndrome: 50 Years' Experience." *Annals of Thoracic Surgery* 86: 254–60.

Valles, S. 2018. *Philosophy of Population Health: Philosophy for a New Public Health Era*. New York: Routledge.

Van Ravenzwaaij, J., T. C. Olde Hartman, H. Van Ravesteijn, R. Eveleigh, E. Van Rijswijk, and P. L. B. J. Lucassen. 2010. "Explanatory Models of Medically Unexplained Symptoms: A Qualitative Analysis of the Literature." *Mental Health in Family Medicine* 7: 223–31.

Watson, J. 2020. *Expertise: A Philosophical Introduction*. New York: Bloomsbury.

Whitney, S. 2003. "A New Model of Medical Decisions: Exploring the Limits of Shared Decision Making." *Medical Decision Making* 23(4): 275–80.

Wilson, C. 1999. "My Years with Lyme Disease." *BMJ* 319: 649.

Wood, P., S. Stanworth, J. Burton, A. Jones, D. G. Peckham, T. Green, C. Hyde, and H. Chapel. 2007. "Recognition, Clinical Diagnosis and Management of Patients with Primary Antibody Deficiencies: A Systematic Review." *Clinical and Experimental Immunology* 149(3): 410–23.

Worrall, J. 2007. "Why There's No Cause to Randomize." *British Journal for Philosophy of Science* 58(3): 451–88.

Yancy, C. 2020. "Academic Medicine and Black Lives Matter: A Time for Deep Listening." *JAMA* 324(5): 435–36. doi:10.1001/jama.2020.12532

Zagury-Orly, I., and R. M. Schwartzstein. 2020. "Covid-19: A Reminder to Reason." Retrieved from https://www.nejm.org/doi/full/10.1056/NEJMp2009405

INDEX

For the benefit of digital users, indexed terms that span two pages (e.g., 52–53) may, on occasion, appear on only one of those pages.